WHAT NURSES KNOW . . .

# CHRONIC FATIGUE SYNDROME

# WHAT NURSES KNOW ...

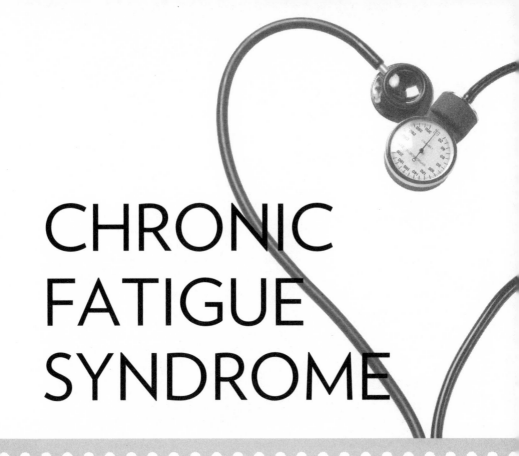

# CHRONIC
# FATIGUE
# SYNDROME

Lorraine Steefel, RN, MSN, DNP, CTN-A

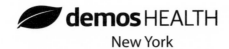

**demos** HEALTH

New York

ISBN: 978-1-932603-87-3
E-ISBN: 978-1-617050-28-2
Visit our web site at www.demoshealth.com

*Acquisitions Editor:* Noreen Henson
*Compositor:* Newgen
*Printer:* Hamilton Printing

Medical information provided by Demos Health, in the absence of a visit with a health care professional, must be considered as an educational service only. This book is not designed to replace a physician's independent judgment about the appropriateness or risks of a procedure or therapy for a given patient. Our purpose is to provide you with information that will help you make your own health care decisions.

The information and opinions provided here are believed to be accurate and sound, based on the best judgment available to the authors, editors, and publisher, but readers who fail to consult appropriate health authorities assume the risk of any injuries. The publisher is not responsible for errors or omissions. The editors and publisher welcome any reader to report to the publisher any discrepancies or inaccuracies noticed.

**Library of Congress Cataloging-in-Publication Data**
Steefel, Lorraine.
    What nurses know-- chronic fatigue syndrome / Lorraine Steefel.
    Summary: "What Nurses Know ... CFS provides validation to the more than one million PWCFS in the United States. It presents an overview of the illness and the latest information about, and description of, symptoms, as well as suggested management of them. It discusses getting a diagnosis and putting together a health care team; for example, readers may choose a neurologist for management of their newly acquired headaches or a rheumatologist for joint pain. Emphasis is placed on the importance of finding a knowledgeable, caring health care provider who is supportive, learning how to communicate with the health care provider and team, and making the most of appointment time"—Provided by publisher.
    Includes index.
    ISBN 978-1-932603-87-3 (pbk.)
    1. Chronic fatigue syndrome—Popular works. I. Title.
    RB150.F37S74 2011
    616'.0478—dc23                                                       2011028540

Made in the United States of America
11  12  13  14  15            5  4  3  2  1

# About the Author

**Lorraine Steefel, RN, MSN, DNP, CTN-A,** is a professional writer and an adjunct professor in the doctoral program at UMDNJ School of Nursing, Newark, NJ. Her interest in CFS developed when her daughter Trisha was diagnosed at age 12 with the illness. As a parent and an RN, she searched for information necessary to help her daughter cope with and manage this illness. She became a volunteer trainer in the program "Chronic Fatigue Syndrome (CFS): A Diagnostic & Management Challenge" prepared and sponsored by the CFIDS Association of America, and presented this program to RNs and other health care professionals across the country. In addition, she is a member of and volunteer for the New Jersey CFS Association. Her fact sheet *Chronic Fatigue Syndrome (ME/CFS) Information for Family, Friends and Caregivers* appears on the organization's website. Lorraine lives in Marlboro Township, NJ, with her husband Peter. She has two daughters, Kimberly and Trisha, and son-in-law, Russ.

## WHAT NURSES KNOW...

Nurses hold a critical role in modern health care that goes beyond their day-to-day duties. They share more information with patients than any other provider group, and are alongside patients twenty-four hours a day, seven days a week, offering understanding of complex health issues, holistic approaches to ailments, and advice for the patient that extends to the family. Nurses themselves are a powerful tool in the healing process.

*What Nurses Know* gives down-to-earth information, addresses consumers as equal partners in their care, and explains clearly what readers need to know and want to know to understand their condition and move forward with their lives.

*Titles published in the series*

**What Nurses Know...PCOS**
Karen Roush

**What Nurses Know...Menopause**
Karen Roush

**What Nurses Know...Diabetes**
Rita Girouard Mertig

**What Nurses Know...Multiple Sclerosis**
Carol Saunders

**What Nurses Know...Gluten-Free Lifestyle**
Sylvia Llewelyn Bower

**What Nurses Know...Chronic Fatigue Syndrome**
Lorraine Steefel

*Forthcoming books in the series*

**What Nurses Know...HIV and AIDS**
Rose Farnan and Maithe Enrigue

**What Nurses Know...PTSD**
Mary Muscari

This book is dedicated to my daughter Trisha, whose journey through CFS inspired me to write. I would also like to thank the New Jersey Chronic Fatigue Syndrome Association, Inc. (NJCFSA) and its members who have shared their stories. Their courage and continued perseverance to get on with life despite—and with—symptoms that vary in intensity day to day, hour to hour, and minute to minute have touched me deeply. Because of this organization, I was provided with many of the tools necessary to support Trisha when she was diagnosed at the age of 12 with CFS.

# Contents

Foreword    *xi*

Introduction    *xiii*

**1**    What Is CFS?    *1*

**2**    Getting a Diagnosis    *15*

**3**    CFS Symptoms    *25*

**4**    Your Health Care Team    *37*

**5**    Save Energy, Keep up With Living,
       Prevent Postexertional Malaise    *51*

**6**    Feelings, Mood Swings, and Depression    *65*

**7**    Medical Treatments for Chronic Fatigue Syndrome    *75*

**8**    Alternative Approaches    *85*

**9**    The Importance of Advocacy    *97*

**10**    Looking Ahead: Living With Chronic Illness    *111*

Glossary    *121*

Resources    *129*

Bibliography    *143*

Index    *163*

# Foreword

Lorraine Steefel has penned an informative, well-written, and well-researched book worth reading by anyone affected by chronic fatigue syndrome (CFS) and those who know and love them. As a nurse and parent of a person dealing with CFS, she is uniquely qualified to write about the personal as well as medical aspects of this chronic illness. The first two chapters explain the syndrome and how it is diagnosed, which should help anyone interested in getting a better understanding of the illness as well as the difficulty and frustration with obtaining a diagnosis. The vignettes in each chapter bring home the various aspects that help the reader relate to the information presented.

As a nurse-author and a person living with a chronic disease myself, I especially liked the chapters concerning the importance of a supportive health care team, alternative and complementary therapies, and advocacy. The advice in Chapter 4 should be especially useful to caregivers who provide aid to those with CFS to seek balance in their own lives. Chapters 5 and 6 provide useful guidance in living with this often unpredictable syndrome, and Chapter 7 lists and explains the various current medical treatments for CFS.

When someone experiences an illness with symptoms as varied and changeable as those of CFS, it is helpful to read about the possibilities and be prepared to seek medical care in a timely manner if and when they occur. The research presented in this book should help health care practitioners to better understand the symptoms these clients experience, the many tests useful in ruling in or ruling out their connection to CFS, and providing appropriate care. Above all, these health care professionals should be encouraged to give respect and understanding the clients with this syndrome and their families deserve.

This book will shed some light on this chronic illness, of which 80 percent of those affected remain undiagnosed, according to the Centers for Disease Control and Prevention. People with CFS may recognize some of the symptoms described, be encouraged to seek help, and work toward turning their life around. Steefel has a proactive and positive approach to a complex and confusing syndrome. As Steefel states in this book, life is a balancing act. Through trial and error, clients with CFS must discover what works and what does not; what to avoid or minimize and when; how to ask for and get the help they need; and how this chronic illness affects them individually so they can improve their quality of life.

Rita Girouard Mertig, MS, RNC, CNS, DE
Author of *What Nurses Know...Diabetes*
(Demos Health, 2011) and the *Nurses' Guide to Teaching Diabetes Self-Management, 2nd ed.*
(Springer Publishing Company, 2012)

# Introduction

In the mid-1980s, I read a magazine article about groups of people in Lake Tahoe, NV, and Lyndonville, NY, who were coming down with a flu-like illness that left them extremely fatigued. They were so fatigued, they couldn't go to work or function the way they did before becoming ill. The article referred to it as the "yuppie flu" because the majority who reported the illness were young, upwardly mobile (YUPPIE), and from the middle class. At that time, people with fatigue, muscle pain, and depression were often diagnosed with chronic Epstein–Barr virus or chronic mononucleosis, so the illness took on these names and was eventually called chronic fatigue syndrome (CFS). Although the cause remained unknown, the illness remained a mystery.

I put down the article and wondered what this new illness was. What caused it? Would I ever contract it? Little did I know that years later, in 1995 to be exact, I would come face to face with it when our daughter Trish was diagnosed with CFS.

Flash forward fifteen years, after helping our daughter deal with CFS and learn how to manage it, I've written *What Nurses Know...CFS* for people with CFS (PWCFS) and their families and friends to provide information drawn from research and reputable sources on the illness. This information is what patients need to know and want to know about their illness and move forward with their lives.

In an effort to make CFS "real" to readers, I've included true-to-life vignettes that describe some aspect of CFS as told to me by PWCFS, as well as examples of what our daughter has experienced living with a chronic illness. These demonstrate what it is like to live, manage, and cope with CFS. They demonstrate that CFS is not an "all in your head" illness. Indeed, in 2006, the U.S. Centers for Disease Control and Prevention began a campaign of awareness that CFS is a real illness, and released brief guidelines encouraging physicians to consider CFS in symptomatic patients when other illnesses are ruled out.

*What Nurses Know...CFS* provides validation to the more than one million PWCFS in the United States. It presents an overview of the illness and the latest information about, and description of, symptoms, as well as suggested management of them. It discusses getting a diagnosis and putting together a health care team; for example, readers may choose a neurologist for management of their newly acquired headaches or a rheumatologist for joint pain. Emphasis is placed on the importance of finding a knowledgeable, caring health care provider who is supportive, learning how to communicate with the health care provider and team, and making the most of appointment time.

Living with CFS is challenging. The book addresses coping with CFS physically and emotionally. Pacing oneself is one suggestion that addresses postexertional malaise (which can result from overextending oneself) and provides a basis for keeping up with daily living activities. Unique to this book are useful thoughts from PWCFS regarding what helped them with a specific symptom or how to cope when things got tough.

Special attention is paid to how important it is for PWCFS to take care of themselves rather than trying to keep up with the crowd. For example, the "no pain, no gain" philosophy typical among the U.S. population is harmful for PWCFS and can cause the illness to flare up. Complementary and alternative medicine as well as integrative therapies are discussed as approaches that can be an effective part of a healing approach for care.

Self-advocacy is a major issue for PWCFS, who must learn to stand up for themselves and their needs, and have the knowledge and the courage to request specific services that will improve their quality of life. The debilitating symptoms of CFS can make it difficult and sometimes impossible to navigate through the employment, education, or health care systems; therefore, having the right people as advocates can make a significant difference.

The book is user friendly, so people can easily access the information they want and need without having to wade through unnecessarily complex data or details. For this reason, it contains bulleted lists; definitions of common terms; and resources such as lists of support groups, Web sites, and online tools.

Chronic fatigue syndrome is a chronic illness, meaning the person will not "grow out of it." It is an up-and-down illness that demands attention and care lest the PWCFS have a flare-up. *What Nurses Know...CFS,* written by a nurse–parent of an individual with CFS, is meant to guide and assist PWCFS live the best quality of life possible and provide information to caregivers and loved ones who assist them on their journey.

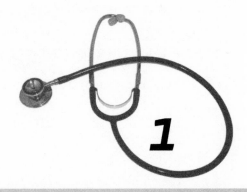

# What Is CFS?

*Picture an inflated balloon. You are that balloon that develops
a small pinprick so that air begins to escape. You deflate physically, emotionally, mentally, and spiritually so that all that's
left of you is an empty shell. All you want to do is sleep. You
just can't shake the fatigue. For me, fatigue is the worst of the
CFS symptoms because you just can't beat it.* LYDIA

## What's in a Name?

Although chronic fatigue syndrome (CFS) was originally named
for its most commonly noted characteristic, fatigue, CFS now
has several names, which are defined in this chapter:

- Chronic fatigue immune dysfunction syndrome
- Myalgic encephalomyelitis/CFS
- CFS/myalgic encephalomyelitis

At publication of this book, the name CFS is still widely used in the media and among research circles in the United States, and therefore, to avoid confusion, this book will refer to the illness as CFS.

Researchers and advocacy groups have attempted to change the name CFS to one that they believe better reflects its nature. Some think that the name CFS can lead to misperceptions that trivialize the illness, for example, people in general complain about how fatigued they may feel at one time or another. The fatigue in CFS is very different. It is intense, overwhelming, cannot be relieved by simple rest, and can be made worse by physical and mental activity. Because CFS encompasses more than fatigue, the search for a name continues.

Some of the other names for CFS are as follows: CFIDS (chronic fatigue immune dysfunction syndrome) as defined by the CFIDS Association of America on the premise that people with CFS (PWCFS) have a defect in the immune system that may predispose them to the illness. Some researchers believe that CFS is an autoimmune disease similar to lupus, but this has proven inconclusive. In many PWCFS, the immune system is affected, resulting in a decrease in immune function.

While research has identified some immune system irregularities, evidence is not yet conclusive that problems with the immune system may be the cause of the symptoms. Interactions among the immune, endocrine, and nervous systems and the role they may play in CFS are under investigation, as well as the various infectious agents and genetic and environmental factors that may be involved in the origins and pathogenesis of the illness.

In countries like Great Britain, CFS is referred to as myalgic encephalomyelitis (ME)/CFS or CFS/ME, while some experts use the terms interchangeably. Myalgic means muscle pain or tenderness. Encephalomyelitis means inflammation of the brain and spinal cord. Some researchers say that E stands for *encephalopathy*, which means altered brain function and struc-ture caused by diffuse brain disease.

In Canada, CFS recently had a name change to ME/CFS. As of April 2010, ME/CFS was officially recognized as a neuro-logic illness by the government of Ontario, Canada, and given the diagnostic code 795. The ground-breaking implications are that people with ME/CFS (in Canada) can never be told by a health care provider that ME/CFS does not exist. This offi-cial recognition will help individuals who apply for disability and pensions in that country. The hope is that other provin-cial ministries of health in Canada (and the world) will soon follow.

In 2007, the CFS/ME Name Change Committee in the United States, consisting of researchers and clinicians, met in Florida, and reached a consensus that the name CFS be changed. The Committee prefers the name ME, saying it is more diagnosti-cally accurate. ME refers to nervous system pathology with associated muscle pain. To avoid problems with insurance and disability claims, the committee recommended that CFS accom-pany ME as part of the name for a period of time.

*Giving a name to your illness is of utmost importance. CFS might be a misnomer, but I'm not sure. What I do know is that the fatigue [in CFS] is the worst symptom. It takes everything out of you. I do know that putting a name to the illness meant that I would no longer be labeled a malingerer by frustrated health care professionals who tried to dismiss me when they couldn't find out what was wrong.*    LYDIA

## In Search of a Definition

To understand and manage an illness, it is necessary to call it by a name that adequately reflects what it is and to construct a defi-nition that clearly explains it. Researchers and advocacy groups continue their work to do this. Here's a glance at historical underpinnings from the late 1980s through the present naming and defining of CFS:

In 1988, experts from the Centers for Disease Control and Prevention (CDC) proposed that the name for chronic Epstein-Barr virus (from the Lake Tahoe and Lyndonville outbreaks) be changed to chronic fatigue syndrome to reflect the major complaint: fatigue. They defined CFS as an illness with two major criteria and at least *eight* symptoms:

- Persistent or relapsing, debilitating fatigue, lasting at least six months, in a person who has no previous history of similar symptoms, and
- Exclusion of other clinical conditions that may produce similar symptoms (e.g., malignancy, autoimmune disease, chronic psychiatric disease, and chronic inflammatory disease, among others)

To be diagnosed with CFS, the person had to have *eight* symptoms, which included mild fever, sore throat, painful lymph nodes, prolonged fatigue after exercise, joint or muscle pain, unexplained muscle weakness, headaches, and sleep disturbance.

About this time, researchers from Australia and Great Britain devised their own definitions of CFS. Australia accepted the CDC definition and added the symptoms of difficulties with short-term memory and concentration. Great Britain developed the Oxford criteria of CFS symptoms and defined postinfectious fatigue syndrome, a subtype of CFS that either follows an infection or is associated with a current infection.

In 1994, the International Chronic Fatigue Syndrome Study Group, headed by the CDC and including representatives from Australia and Great Britain, drafted a revised case definition of CFS, which is the one most widely used today. Named after Keiji Fukuda, the first author of the manuscript in which it is

*What Nurses Know . . .*
● ● ● ● ● ● ● ● ● ● ● ● ● ● ● ● ● ● ● ● ● ● ● ● ● ●

*The severity of CFS, and how it affects people, varies from person to person. Some are able to lead fairly active lives. By definition, CFS significantly limits work, school, and family activities.*

published, the Fukuda definition is the accepted standard for research studies. Health care providers use this definition to diagnose CFS. According to the Fukuda case definition, to receive a diagnosis of CFS a person must have

1. severe chronic fatigue of six months or longer with other known medical conditions excluded by clinical diagnosis; and
2. four or more of the following symptoms concurrently (within the six-month time frame):
   - substantial impairment in short-term memory or concentration
   - sore throat
   - tender lymph nodes
   - muscle pain
   - multi-joint pain without swelling or redness
   - headaches of a new type, pattern, or severity
   - unrefreshing sleep
   - postexertional malaise lasting more than 24 hours

## Defining Continues

Because the 1994 (Fukuda) case definition was developed with adults in mind, researchers called together a Working Group for a pediatric definition of CFS. In 2006, the International

Association of Chronic Fatigue Syndrome (now called the International Association of CFS/ME) published the *Pediatric Case Definition for Myalgic Encephalomyelitis and Chronic Fatigue Syndrome.* As part of meeting the diagnostic criteria for CFS within this pediatric definition, children and adolescents must have experienced fatigue and symptoms for at least three months, rather than the six-month criteria as with adults. The pediatric case definition includes a comprehensive questionnaire that doctors and other professionals can use to specifically assess CFS in children.

Although the 1994 CFS (Fukuda) case definition is widely used in the United States today, in 2003, researchers and clinicians from the United States and other nations developed another case definition for the illness, *Myalgic Encephalomyelitis/Chronic Fatigue Syndrome: Clinical Working Definition, Diagnostic and Treatment Protocols.* This definition, published partially under the auspices of the Canadian Ministry of Health, is informally called the Canadian definition. It combines the findings from the CDC-sponsored research on CFS and the European research on ME.

## DEFINITIONS OF CFS AND CLINICAL GUIDELINES

Because CFS has no known cause or cure, considerable debate continues regarding how to accurately define the illness. The CFS International (Fukuda) definition remains the accepted standard for research, which health care providers use to diagnose patients. The following are definitions and clinical guidelines as they were developed and published.

- CFS–The CDC definition (1988)
- CFS–The Australian definition (1990)
- CFS–The British definition (1991)
- CFS–The international definition (1994)
- The international CFS definition revisited (2003)

## What Nurses Know . . .

*Because the cause of CFS is still unknown, health care providers rely on a CFS case definition to help them diagnose the illness. The case definition encourages a diagnosis based on characteristic patterns of patients' symptoms.*

- ME/CFS–The Canadian Clinical Case Definition (2003). http://www.cfids-cab.org/MESA/ccpccd.pdf
- ME/CFS guidelines (2004 Clinical Guidelines form Australia). http://www.cfids-cab.org/MESA/AU_CFS.pdf
- ME/CFS: Delay harms health, early diagnosis: why is it so important? A report from the ME Alliance (UK) (2005). http://www.cfids-cab.org/MESA/EarlyDiagnosis.pdf
- Pediatric Case Definition for ME/CFS. Jason, L. A., Bell, D. S., De Meirleir, K., et al. (2006). *Journal of Chronic Fatigue Syndrome, 13*(2/3), 1-44. http://www.cfids-cab.org/MESA/Jason-1a.pdf
- Assessment and treatment of patients with ME/CFS: Clinical guidelines for psychiatrists. Stein, Eleanor, MD, FRCP(C). http://www.cfids-cab.org/MESA/Stein.pdf
- A case definition for children with ME/CFS. Jason, L. A., Porter, N., Shelleby, E., Bell, D. S., Lapp, C. W., Rowe, K., De Meirleir, K. (2008). *Clinical Medicine: Pediatrics, 1*, 53-57. http://www.cfids-cab.org/MESA/Jason-1b.pdf

## A Symptom-Defined Illness

My daughter Trish had more than four of the symptoms, including the overwhelming fatigue that researchers described. No matter how much sleep she got, she was still tired. Her pediatrician found the tender axillary lymph nodes and the characteristic crimson-colored arc in the back of her very sore throat. Different joints or muscles hurt her on different days, and she used braces for her elbows, knees, or ankles and elastic bandages for achy muscles. Trish developed migraine headaches that pounded on the top of her head, often accompanied by a swollen area we called a bump on the top of her skull. At times, she seemed as if she were living in a fog and had difficulty concentrating or thinking of the appropriate word she wanted to say.

The physician who diagnosed Trish relied on her account of the symptoms that she experienced because there were, and still are, no tests to diagnose CFS. Reliance on subjective symptoms rather than tests for diagnosis is one of the reasons why CFS is considered an illness rather than a disease.

Scientists are moving closer to finding the pathogenesis of CFS, that is, what goes wrong in the body to cause such an array of symptoms. Once they find this, CFS might then be considered a "disease" as opposed to a "syndrome." So far, researchers have identified abnormalities in the brain (central nervous system) and the immune system, providing evidence that the illness involves and alters the function of these two systems. For

*The fog is what has always scared me the most. I remember once when I was 16 and living in the only home I'd ever known, I forgot where the toilet paper was. And I don't mean that we had run out. I didn't just forget if there was more under the sink or above the washing machine. I mean I was sitting on the toilet and literally could not remember how to reach for the toilet paper. Was it to my left? To my right? I got so exasperated and was so afraid, I started to cry. I remember thinking, "This is what Nana (my senile grandmother) must feel like."* TRISH example, it is believed that low levels of the hormone cortisol could activate the immune system and result in brain dysfunction. This could lead to fatigue, cognitive dysfunction, pain sensitivity, and other symptoms.

Some studies have shown that CFS began after a viral illness. Some researchers of CFS study a possible link between CFS and EBV, the cause of mononucleosis. Some believe that EBV (and other infectious agents) or their reactivation can trigger CFS in people who are genetically predisposed to it, but more research is needed to confirm the links. It is possible that in CFS, different infectious agents interact to cause symptoms.

While many experts believe that CFS is linked to one or more infectious agents, like viruses, CFS is not contagious in the typical sense that you can "catch" it from someone. Although there have been at least three reported community "outbreaks" in the past twenty-five years, most have been isolated cases within the communities.

Researchers are looking for biomarkers, for example, proteins that show up in greater quantities in the blood of PWCFS, in order to create diagnostic tests for CFS. In 2011, CFS gained media attention when researchers at six institutions led by UMDNJ (University of Medicine and Dentistry of NJ) reported finding protein markers in the spinal fluid of PWCFS that distinguished them from people with Lyme disease, which has some similar symptoms, and healthy controls. The encouraging news from these findings is that this new data can be analyzed in the search to develop the cause or pathogenesis of CFS. As lead researcher for UMDNJ, Steven E. Schutzer says, "The next step is to narrow down the list of proteins to find the best biomarkers for what is going wrong in the central nervous system."

Some have speculated on an environmental component, such as toxic exposure, as a possible cause of CFS, but this has yet to be proven. CFS appears to be triggered by a stressor of some kind, but this is not necessary. The apparent stressor is typically physiologic, such as a viral infection or toxic exposure,

**INFECTIOUS AGENTS LINKED TO CFS**

- *EBV*
- *Post Q fever* (Coxiella burnetti)
- *Ross River virus*
- *Lyme* (B. burdorferi) *(yes, but unusual)*
- *Parvovirus (yes, but unusual)*
- *Enteroviruses*
- *Human herpesvirus-6*
- *Xenotropic murine leukemia virus-related virus*
- *Other murine leukemia retroviruses*

but may be a mental or physical trauma that leads to CFS many years later. As yet, no single causative agent of CFS has yet been identified.

Rather than pointing a finger at the infectious agent as the cause, some researchers believe that CFS is the result of an abnormality in the way the body responds to the infectious agent. The immune system continues to fight off the infectious agent when it is no longer there.

People may use the words illness and disease interchangeably, but they are different. A disease has a known cause, and may have a diagnostic test, a cure, and a predictable course in the way it affects people. The disease tuberculosis (TB), for example, is caused by a pathogen, the bacterium *Mycobacterium tuberculosis*, and is treated with antibiotics. Tests of patients' sputum can detect TB. Its signs and symptoms, clinical course, treatment, and prognosis are similar in the people it affects across the globe.

PWCFS experience periods of illness and relative wellness, with symptoms that change over time. Some grow progressively worse; others recover completely or improve enough to return to activities but still experience CFS symptoms. According to the CFIDS Association of America, the majority of PWCFS seem to improve within five years of becoming ill. Based on statistical data from the CDC, if symptoms last for five years, it is unlikely that the illness will improve significantly in subsequent years.

As its name suggests, CFS is also referred to as a syndrome, a collection of signs and symptoms known to frequently appear together but without a known cause. The word syndrome may tempt people to dismiss the seriousness of CFS and think, "Oh, it's just a syndrome." However, the National Institutes of Health describes CFS as a debilitating complex syndrome that involves multiple body systems. Persons with CFS most often function much below the activity levels they enjoyed before its onset.

## Who Gets CFS?

If you are the person who contracts CFS, you put a human face on this illness. Since mid-2006, a CFS photo exhibit "The Faces of Chronic Fatigue Syndrome" sponsored by the CFIDS Association of America has told the stories of PWCFS: a mother and daughter, a twelve-year-old boy former athlete and academic achiever, a young man in college, a young mother with three children, a Vietnam Veteran, and more. It has traveled to more than forty venues across the country, showing the personal meanings behind the statistics.

Although numbers as such don't count for those who are struggling with the exhaustion, pain, cognitive dysfunction, and other symptoms, numbers are helpful because they remind PWCFS that they are not alone. Statistics help to legitimize a real illness and assist researchers in their work to understand and help find the cause and cure.

The CDC says between one and four million people in the United States have CFS, with almost twenty percent having symptoms but remaining undiagnosed. The CFIDS Association of American says that CFS strikes more people in the United States than multiple sclerosis, lupus, lung cancer, or AIDS.

CFS is sometimes seen in members of the same family. Researchers are studying the possibility of a familial or genetic link to the risk of developing CFS. There may be genetic factors that predispose someone to get CFS. Research into the genes themselves has led to the identification of eighty-eight genes whose genetic expression differs significantly in CFS patients compared with healthy people in control groups. (Genetic expression refers to the products that genes produce, typically proteins.) Research in London led by Dr. Jonathan Kerr has found that there are seven likely genomic subtypes. These subtypes correlate with clusters of different types of CFS symptoms and with how severe the symptoms are. Each genomic subtype is believed to be a distinct condition.

CFS can affect people of all ethnic and socioeconomic backgrounds. Although some studies say that rates are higher in Hispanics, African Americans, and those with lower socioeconomic status, larger epidemiologic studies are required to confirm these findings. Research indicates that CFS is at least as common among African Americans and Hispanics as it is among whites.

Although no one knows why, statistically more women than men, with a ratio of 4 to 1, appear to contract CFS, but that does not place CFS into a category as a "woman's disease." Noted Australian infectious diseases specialist Andrew Lloyd and colleagues say that CFS has nothing to do with gender, age, personality type, or mental health. CFS is most commonly triggered by an acute illness, like glandular fever, and it is the severity of this illness that determines whether someone will develop the syndrome. "The sicker you are at the beginning of the infection, the more likely it is to result in a prolonged illness," says Dr. Lloyd.

The majority of people are diagnosed with CFS in their forties and fifties, but children and adolescents can develop the illness. It is difficult to determine how many children have CFS because there was no pediatric definition used to diagnose them until 2006. Pediatric CFS can range in severity from mild to moderate

(moderate symptoms at rest that become severe with effort, unable to attend school) to severe (often completely housebound or bedbound). Although CFS is the same illness in adults and in children, the symptoms and course of the illness can vary.

## Is CFS Contagious?

There is no evidence that CFS is contagious; however, researchers believe that infectious agents may trigger and perpetuate CFS and that the infectious agents cannot be fully eradicated by the immune system. Also, CFS can follow a new infection, such as after Lyme disease.

The National Cancer Institute and CFS Advocacy organizations like the CFIDS Association of America have historically discouraged PWCFS from donating blood or organs, based on safety concerns for both the donor and the receiver. PWCFS have low blood volume and orthostatic intolerance (dizziness related to low blood volume). They have frequent infections that may or may not be passed on to receivers.

The AABB (formerly the American Association of Blood Banking) recommends that blood collectors actively discourage potential donors who have been diagnosed with CFS from donating blood. This response was made after the publication of a paper in the journal *Science* that reported the discovery of xenotropic murine leukemia virus–related virus (XMRV), a retrovirus previously linked to prostate cancer, in 67% of 101 patients with CFS, and 4% of 218 in the healthy control group. Although the findings have not been repeated in the European research community, and conflicting data are a cause to warrant more research, concerns were raised about a possible role for XMRV in CFS. More research is being conducted. In the meantime, not donating blood or organs mitigates the possible risk of transmission of XMRV. The recommendations have been implemented by the American Red Cross and America's Blood Centers.

## What Nurses Know ...

• • • • • • • • • • • • • • • • • • • • • • • • • • • •

*Eighty percent of PWC remain undiagnosed. An early diagnosis of CFS means that treatment of symptoms can begin sooner, leading to a better quality of life.*

## When to Seek Treatment

If someone has symptoms of CFS, they could have this medical condition or another illness that shares many symptoms of CFS. They should not delay seeking a diagnosis. Although it took almost one year for Trish to be diagnosed with CFS, there is now greater awareness of CFS among the medical community that generally means an earlier diagnosis and earlier management of symptoms.

Like any chronic condition, learning about CFS is of utmost importance. Any chronic illness can affect an individual's friends and family. Family education and seeing a therapist may foster good communication and reduce the adverse effect of CFS on the family.

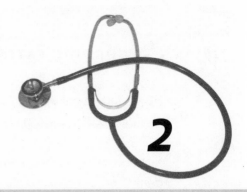

**2**

# Getting a Diagnosis

*It was August 13, 1987, when my 12-year-old son Scott and I thought we had come down with the flu. One day we were fine, and the next day we woke up with an overwhelming fatigue, sore throat, swollen lymph nodes, nausea, and vomiting. I was always athletic, but could barely lift my head off the pillow, let alone get out of bed. Scott was equally as weak and too sick to go to school.*

*Scott's blood work was normal so the pediatrician said that Scott was probably school-phobic. After my husband and I insisted that these symptoms weren't normal for Scott, he referred Scott to an infectious disease specialist who ordered more tests. Results showed elevated levels for the Cytomegalic virus, reduced CD4 and CD8 lymphocyte blood cell counts, and slightly elevated levels for Epstein–Barr virus (EBV). Although these blood tests aren't definitive diagnostic tests, the specialist determined the diagnosis as chronic EBV (the name for CFS at the time). The pediatrician, who didn't "believe" in chronic EBV disagreed, so we were on own to find someone who did.*

*I experienced similar hesitation from my general practitioner until I recounted my son's illness. The physician sent me for additional tests that showed similar results.*

*Finally, we knew what we were dealing with, chronic EBV. Having a name to call this illness validated us. It meant we could look it up to learn more about it, and search for a health care provider who believed in it (and us). It meant we weren't alone. Most of all, it was an extreme relief to know I wouldn't die before I found out what's wrong with me.*   BETTY

## Problems With Diagnosis

People with chronic fatigue syndrome (PWCFS) have unique stories that explain how they were diagnosed with the illness. Betty and her son had an onset of acute symptoms that brought them to health care providers, but it still took some time for them to receive a diagnosis. Unlike Betty and Scott, not all PWCFS experience a sudden onset of the illness; rather they have a more gradual development of symptoms, and become ill.

Also, unlike Betty, some people with chronic fatigue syndrome (CFS) find health care providers knowledgeable about the illness, while others still meet with hesitancy or even resistance to diagnose and/or treat it. In 2006, the Centers for Disease Control and Prevention (CDC) launched the first-ever CFS public awareness campaign, *Get Informed. Get Diagnosed. Get Treated*, to educate the American Public and health care professionals about CFS and call attention to the need for communication between them, facilitating diagnosis and treatment.

## What Nurses Know...

*Here are some factors that make diagnosing CFS challenging:*

- *There is no diagnostic laboratory test or biomarker found in the blood for CFS*
- *Fatigue and other symptoms of CFS are shared by many illnesses*
- *Symptoms vary from person to person in type, number, and severity*
- *No two CFS patients have exactly the same symptoms*
- *CFS has a pattern of remission and relapse*
- *People with CFS don't look ill*

CFS remains a diagnostic and management challenge because CFS has no characteristic clinical signs or laboratory biomarkers in the blood, making diagnosis dependent on self-reported symptoms and ruling out other causes of illness. Fatigue, the overarching symptom, and many of its other symptoms are common to other illnesses. Also, CFS symptoms can disappear and then return and vary from person to person, with no two people having exactly the same symptoms. Little wonder that the CDC estimates that less than 20% of the one million people with CFS have been diagnosed.

## A Rule-Out Illness

Symptoms are meant to alert you that something may be wrong. They are warnings to seek medical attention to get diagnosed and treated with the hope of preventing complications or a serious, even life-threatening event. Some symptoms can look like you have CFS. When patients have fatigue, health care providers investigate whether it is caused by CFS or a disease that mimics CFS. Some illnesses that cause fatigue include

- autoimmune illnesses like lupus
- anorexia and bulimia
- bipolar disorder
- cancer
- cardiovascular disease
- diabetes
- endometriosis
- Gulf war syndrome
- hepatitis
- hypothyroidism
- multiple sclerosis

You can see, just from this list, that fatigue goes hand in hand with many conditions and diseases.

Making the diagnosis even more complicated, conditions like fibromyalgia (FM) share symptoms with CFS, such as fatigue and pain, and also lack a diagnostic test or biomarker. However, before health care providers can consider CFS for a diagnosis, they must rule out these and other diseases through medical testing. You may wonder why your health care provider is sending you for "so many tests." These are necessary in the journey toward diagnosis.

Step 1 for health care providers is to take a thorough history from patients, and then conduct a physical examination and screening of the mental status of patients. In their search for a diagnosis, providers should prescribe a variety of laboratory tests, such as the following that are suggested by the CDC in their *CFS Toolkit*:

- Urinalysis
- Total protein

- Glucose C-reactive protein
- Phosphorus electrolyte
- Complete blood count with leukocyte differential
- Alkaline phosphatase
- Creatinine
- Blood urea nitrogen
- Albumin
- ANA
- Rheumatoid factor
- Globulin
- Calcium
- Alanine
- Aminotransferase
- Aspartate transminase serum level
- Thyroid function tests (thyroid-stimulating hormone and Free T4)

Health care providers may also prescribe further tests or provide referrals to specialists to confirm or exclude a diagnosis that better explains the fatigue, or to follow-up on results of the

## What Nurses Know...

*The CFIDS Association of America online questionnaire can help patients look at their symptoms objectively to see if they fit with the general pattern of CFS symptoms. Although the questionnaire is not meant to substitute for a medical assessment and is not meant to discourage people from seeking medical attention for diagnosis, it can help people understand whether or not they have CFS. The questionnaire can be found at their Web site.*

initial tests. Those other or concurrent illnesses would then be treated.

## Case Definition + Symptoms + Rule-Out Illnesses

The blood tests that Betty and her son had were not specific tests used to diagnose CFS; rather, they were used to identify abnormalities that could be related to CFS. After the results of all tests are in, health care providers rule out any other possible cause for their patients' illness and consider the symptoms they are having. According to the CDC, they refer to the CFS case definition to determine whether patients fit the criteria and give a diagnosis of CFS when no cause for the symptoms is identified and if the other conditions of the case definition are met.

At the time of diagnosis, Betty and Scott had overwhelming fatigue for more than six months that severely altered their quality of life. They also demonstrated four or more of the symptoms within that time frame: difficulty concentrating, sore throat, headache, enlarged lymph nodes, muscle and/or joint pain, and postexertional malaise (feelings of illness for 24 hours after exertion of energy). They fit the CDC case definition of CFS.

## *What Nurses Know . . .*

*It is a myth that CFS is defined just by a group of symptoms with no objective abnormalities. Researchers have found abnormalities in several of the systems of the body of PWCFS—the central, autonomic nervous, and immune systems. These abnormalities are not present in people who are healthy or who have other fatiguing illnesses.*

## Watch Out for Overlapping and Related Conditions

Some people with CFS have other illnesses that health care providers should be on the look out for to diagnose and treat. These overlapping conditions are called comorbidities. Morbid means sickness or induced by disease. Comorbidity refers to the presence of one or more disorders or diseases in addition to a primary disease. These comorbid conditions are medical problems that often occur with CFS. Researchers are studying genes and environmental factors as possible factors that influence syndromes like CFS with symptoms such as chronic widespread pain, chronic fatigue, irritable bowel syndrome, and recurrent headache.

Based on high rates of cooccurrence and overlapping diagnosis criteria, some researchers propose that CFS, FM, and multiple chemical sensitivity (MCS) are the same illness, while others distinguish them from each other. Needless to say,

*What Nurses Know . . .*

*CFS and many of its overlapping conditions disproportionately affect women. According to the Campaign to End Chronic Pain in Women, formed by the Overlapping Conditions Alliance, as many as fifty million women live with one or more neglected chronic pain conditions (pain for more than six months) such as CFS, interstitial cystitis, fibromyalgia, temporomandibular joint disorder (TMJ), vulvodynia, and endometriosis. The Campaign aims to improve the quality of women's lives by raising awareness of these chronic pain conditions and to the neglect, dismissal, and discrimination faced by women suffering from chronic pain.*

having more than one illness compounds the diagnostic challenge and impacts the person's symptoms and related disability. Researchers have found that people with CFS, FM, and MCS have more pain, fatigue, sleep disturbances, depression, and poorer physical functioning than those who had CFS alone.

While there has been great debate about how to define or diagnose CFS, criteria have been established. If your doctor does not "believe" in CFS, get a second opinion. The earlier a person with CFS receives medical treatment, the greater the likelihood that the illness will resolve.

People being treated for overlapping conditions alongside CFS should talk to their health care providers about possible

## What Nurses Know . . .

*Research has shown that some people with CFS have disturbances in the regulation of their blood pressure called neurally mediated hypotension, which can cause dizziness and even fainting. They should avoid standing for prolonged periods—or when in warm places such as a hot shower—to avoid triggering these events.*

## What Nurses Know . . .

*For people with CFS, multiple medical problems are generally the rule, not the exception. This makes diagnosis more difficult and time consuming, but all the more necessary. Treating overlapping conditions may help to alleviate some of the CFS symptoms. Treating them and the symptoms of CFS as soon as possible lessens the possibility of becoming worse.*

medication interactions. For example, someone taking selective serotonin reuptake inhibitor or serotonin-norepinephrine reuptake inhibitor antidepressants should not also take tricyclic antidepressants, which are typically used for interstitial cystitis.

As always, it is important to continue routine health care checkups and tests such as screening mammograms, pap smears, cholesterol blood work, blood pressure screenings. PWCFS may forget to do so because they may feel too ill to schedule healthy checkups. This can lead to missing a potential health problem not related to CFS.

## What's Next?

As Betty's story shows, having a diagnosis is meaningful. It dispels the myth that what people with CFS have is "all in their heads." Being able to call the illness by its name gives people a sense that there is something they can fight or manage.

When my daughter Trish was diagnosed, the physician said, "I have good news, and I have bad news." The good news was that he had a name for the illness. "We know what you have, CFS," he said. "The bad news is that we don't have a cure."

We left the doctor's office with mixed feelings. Trish was relieved that she wasn't *crazy*; what she experienced was real. The question that surfaced was, what do we do next?

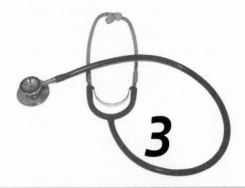

# CFS Symptoms

*I felt as if I had glass in the back of my throat. It hurt like it never hurt before. The pain was so bad I went to the emergency room. The doctors didn't find anything wrong with me and sent me home.* LYDIA

The symptoms of chronic fatigue syndrome (CFS) are unpredictable and can vary from week to week, even hour to hour. CFS affects many of the body's systems, for example, the nervous, immune, cardiovascular, and endocrine systems, where symptoms can originate. In the aforementioned extract, Lydia describes just one symptom people with CFS (PWCFS) have exhibited.

As its name suggests, fatigue is CFS's overarching symptom, but fatigue can mean different things to the many PWCFS. At times, fatigue means brain fog that affects the ability to recall words or remember things. PWCFS may feel mentally confused.

Think of a time when you were physically exhausted, for example, and even thinking was too much work. After mild activity or even no activity at all, fatigue can overwhelm the person with CFS. This postexertional malaise can make you feel like you have the flu. At times, you can feel "wired," that is, you feel overstimulated but lack the energy to do anything in response to this overstimulation, or just lack the energy to carry on normal daily functions.

Symptoms affect people differently in severity and the length of time they last. Not every person experiences each symptom. The following is a list of symptoms included in the diagnostic criteria and a description of what each can feel like to the person with CFS.

- Substantial difficulties with short-term memory or concentration (see cognitive dysfunction described later)—PWCFS can have memory loss that includes constantly forgetting simple information like names and numbers. They seem to have an inability to take in information, may have to read the same thing over and over, have difficulty organizing their thoughts, and complain of feeling like they are in a fog.
- Sore throat—The type of sore throat PWCFS have can result from swollen throat tissue that makes it very difficult to swallow. The resulting pain can be burning and persistent, and can feel as sharp as glass.
- Tender lymph nodes—Soreness of lymph nodes under the arms can range from tenderness to pain that makes it difficult for PWCFS to completely put their arms down at their sides.
- Muscle pain—This pain can feel like unrelievable heaviness, soreness, weakness, or acute pain anywhere in the body.
- Multijoint pain without swelling or redness—This pain most commonly occurs in the lower back and legs but can occur anywhere in the body. The aching can be severe and is aggravated by any physical or even mental exertion.
- Headaches of a new type, pattern, or severity—These headaches feel like intense pressure and can manifest as migraines.

- Unrefreshing sleep—PWCFS feel as if they have not slept at all even after a "good" night's sleep. Sleep disturbances are common and may include either hypersomnolence (sleeping more than normal), insomnia, or sleep reversal (sleeping all day and awake at night).

- Postexertional malaise (postexertional relapse) lasting more than 24 hours—This extreme, prolonged exhaustion is the result of a worsening of symptoms that follow any kind of physical or mental exertion (not necessarily from intense or strenuous activity). It is an inappropriate loss of physical and/or mental stamina compared with the levels of activity leading to it. In fact, the pre-malaise activity would have been easily tolerated before the development of CFS. Postexertional malaise may begin immediately after the activity, or after a period of delay, and may last days or weeks. PWCFS cannot reliably predict what activity might bring it on or how long it will take to recover.

In response to a CFIDS Association of America survey, 1,200 *CFIDSLink* readers, donors, and members of the organization (most of whom were women, most of them aged forty-one to fifty-five, and on average had been ill for more than five years) described what their symptoms were. For all age groups, the most common symptoms were postexertion fatigue, unrefreshing sleep, muscle pain, and concentration problems, followed by joint pain, sinus problems, eye sensitivity to light, depression, and other sleep issues. Less common symptoms seemed to vary by age; for example, pelvic pain was more common in younger people whereas urinary urgency was more common in older adults. Older survey responders ranked the less common symptoms as more severe; however, unrefreshing sleep decreased slightly in this group.

Despite these symptoms, some PWCFS maintain a fairly active life, whereas others are severely debilitated. Symptoms

## What Nurses Know...

*The number and severity of symptoms vary between PWCFS but the core symptoms are listed in the diagnostic criteria. All symptoms are generally made worse by physical or mental exertion of any kind. PWCFS often experience periods of remission and relapse.*

typically follow a cyclical course, alternating between periods of illness and relative well-being. Although some have a partial or complete remission of symptoms during the course of CFS, symptoms often recur and limit work, school, and quality of life. This pattern makes CFS hard for patients to manage, and difficult for health care providers trying to diagnose the illness.

## Other Physical Symptoms

In addition to the symptoms that are included in the diagnostic criteria for the illness, PWCFS complain of many other symptoms. Again, these secondary symptoms may not affect each person with CFS, and they can vary in severity among the affected people. Here are some of the secondary symptoms that PWCFS complain of:

- Dry mouth, eyes
- Canker sores
- Chronic cough
- Periodontal disease, tooth pain
- Impotence
- Swelling of nasal passages, sinusitis
- Tachycardia (fast heart beat), palpitations (skipped heart beats)

- Ringing in the ears
- Nausea
- Fevers/chills/sweats/feeling hot often
- Recurrent illness and infections
- Systemic yeast/fungal infections
- Increased/severe premenstrual syndrome (PMS)
- Sinus pain/swelling of nasal passages

## Neurologic and/or Central Nervous System Symptoms

- Muscle weakness
- Dizziness, spatial disorientation, difficulty standing upright
- Lightheadedness, low blood pressure
- Alcohol intolerance
- Aspartame (artificial sweetener) intolerance
- Memory problems
- Light sensitivity
- Aphasia (difficulty retrieving words)
- Numbness or tingling in extremities
- Confusion, inability to think clearly
- Concentration/attention deficit
- Photosensitivity
- Coordination problems/clumsiness
- Paresthesias (numbness, tingling, or other odd sensations in face and/or extremities)
- Visual disturbance (scratchiness, blurring of vision, "floaters")

## Emotional/Psychological Symptoms

- Anxiety, panic attacks
- Mood swings
- Depression
- Personality changes

Many PWCFS are depressed. According to the *Family Practice Journal,* 36% of individuals with CFS are clinically depressed. PWCFS may wonder which came first, CFS or feeling depressed. With all chronic illnesses, there is a psychological component. We are body, mind, and spirit, and therefore what affects our body will impact our entire person. Feeling physically ill can lead to feelings of depression. We can feel frustrated because we are not our "old" self or our health care providers do not believe there is anything physically wrong. It is important to seek counseling for help with coping and to distinguish between feeling depression due to CFS and a depressive illness that needs particular attention, perhaps medication and/or counseling unique to depression.

> *My sister Cheryl and I have had CFS for years, with many different symptoms, off and on. I remember the first time my skin began to hurt. My clothes felt too heavy and the smallest amount of pressure felt like pain. So I decided to compare notes with Cheryl and find out if her skin hurt as well. When she answered yes, we knew it was another symptom related to CFS.* LYDIA

## Knowing About Symptoms

It is helpful for PWCFS to read ahead of time about the symptoms that can occur. Rather than causing worry, knowledge about possible symptoms can help PWCFS be prepared to emotionally and physically deal with the new symptom, and seek medical attention as needed. Here are some examples of events that occurred when PWCFS were not aware of symptoms that could—and then did—occur.

When Lydia experienced skin sensitivity, she asked her sister whether she was having the same sensation. Lydia was unaware that what people without CFS feel as pressure, people with the illness feel as pain. In fact, some PWCFS have patches of skin that become very sensitive to the touch. They may experience a burning feeling, which they describe as a crawling sensation.

When my daughter Trisha experienced a new sensation—a stabbing pain in the muscles between her ribs while walking down the steps one day—we were both frightened. It wasn't until some time later and after reading about CFS symptoms that we discovered that this new pain (which could not be attributed to anything else) could be associated with CFS.

Early on after Trish's diagnosis, she began having dizzy spells. One afternoon I received a call from her friend's mother telling me that "Trish was okay but she fainted while waiting on line in a department store." We assumed that she had low blood sugar and made sure that she carried with her a tube of cake frosting, similar to what people with diabetes might carry to prevent drops in blood sugar and consequent fainting. Again, we did not associate fainting with CFS until years later when we discovered that dizziness or fainting while standing, called orthostatic intolerance (OI), can be a related symptom. When PWCFS stand for long periods of time, they experience dizziness and even faint because their blood pools to their legs, which decreases the amount of oxygen to the brain. We also discovered that PWCFS can have postural orthostatic tachycardia syndrome (POTS) characterized by a rapid heart rate while standing.

Health care providers of PWCFS who also have OI may suggest that they increase water intake to at least 2 L daily and increase salt intake to 10 to 15 g each day. This suggestion is individual and age related. In a teenager, sodium retention and increased fluids are prescribed; however, increasing sodium intake, which causes the body to retain water, can be a problem for a middle-aged person. You can get swelling of the extremities and high blood pressure at the same time that you have OI, because OI has to do with the rapid drop in blood pressure when standing. The PWCFS who has heart or blood vessel disease should not increase fluid because the increased fluid and its retention could put an extra strain on the heart, causing serious problems.

Medications like β-blockers can help control rapid heart rate and can stabilize the blood vessels that are reacting so dramatically to a position change. To avoid dizziness and fainting, PWCFS can try not to become overheated and can exercise in a way that minimizes OI. Women with CFS, especially those on their feet for some time, can wear control top panty hose to encourage blood flow and prevent severe drops in blood pressure.

People living with CFS may not know that they could have OI. If you are a PWCFS experiencing dizziness, see a cardiologist for an evaluation. Find out whether there is a significant difference between your blood pressure when you sit down and when you stand up.

> *The three most frequent complaints that I hear from PWCFS are: fatigue, dizziness, and headache, followed by GI issues and muscle pain. They come to the clinic for help to deal with these and be able to function as normal as possible, to attend school or go to work, or return to a somewhat normal life. Treatment related to OI or POTS includes medication that will increase blood volume, a medication called a β-blocker that will slow the increased heart rate (tachycardia), and an antidepressant medication or serotonin reuptake inhibitor (SSRI) to decrease depressive symptoms. There is no magic pill; what works for one doesn't necessarily work for someone else. In addition to medication, a positive attitude along with a focus on increasing fluids throughout the day, eating a healthy diet, and exercising as tolerated can help to alleviate OI and POTS. The number one "no no" is staying in bed all day. It's important to move, however little, even if that is to move from the bed to the couch each day.* COURTNEY TERILLI, RN, BSN, Center for Hypertension

Seeking medical attention for new symptoms provides health care providers with the opportunity to rule out the development of another illness, or at least reassure PWCFS that the symptom is related to CFS. In our case, this would have alleviated some of the distress we experienced.

*What Nurses Know...*

*When a new and different symptom occurs, patients with CFS should not assume that it is just another CFS symptom. It is important that a health care provider rules out a possible new illness.*

## A Word About Pain

"Pain is what the person says it is, and exists whenever he or she says it does," says nurse and noted pain researcher Margo McCaffery. This groundbreaking definition can be applied to PWCFS who have a uniquely personal experience with pain. Only they can describe how they feel. No objective tests exist to measure pain. McCaffery's definition lays the groundwork for the respect that people in pain deserve and the care that must be given even if the health care professional does not and cannot understand the pain described.

CFS is an invisible illness; and PWCFS generally look well. No one can see the pain they experience, and are often told they are making it up. This makes it all the more difficult to diagnose.

Some PWCFS who also have another illness such as fibromyalgia (FM) may find it difficult to tell the difference between pain from CFS or FM. When Trisha experiences a gnawing, exhausting bone pain, she knows it is FM pain. When she takes pain medication, she does get some relief from it, although the pain does not entirely go away. If the pain is deep muscle, it stems from CFS and lasts longer. Again, everyone is different and experiences pain differently. Treatment of pain must therefore be on an individual basis.

According to the CFIDS Association of America, most pain relief therapy begins with over-the-counter medications such as aspirin or acetaminophen (Tylenol) or ibuprofen (Advil). For moderately severe pain, health care providers may prescribe mild narcotics with long-lasting narcotics reserved for severe, unrelenting pain. Because PWCFS are sensitive to medications, starting them at lower doses is recommended. Therapies such as meditation or biofeedback have shown to be helpful in conjunction with medication for pain relief. Some PWCFS benefit from the help of a pain management specialist who will monitor the pain and assist them to find the therapy best suited for them.

## Cognitive Dysfunction (Brain Fog)

When my daughter Trish, diagnosed with CFS at age twelve, was well enough to return to Middle School, none of us realized that CFS would impact her ability to learn. She had difficulty memorizing Spanish vocabulary and at times could not compute simple addition problems or recall words or names of people she knew. She seemed as if she were staring into space, and, at times, confused. This was her way of showing brain fog or cognitive dysfunction that occurs at uncertain times. This is a mental fatigue associated with CFS.

Researchers studying cognitive dysfunction in patients with CFS have discovered that the most prominent finding is that information-processing speed and efficiency are impaired. PWCFS perform more poorly on tasks that require rapid manipulation of information and on complex and time-limited tasks. Learning, new memory, and the ability to remember information while performing mental operations with that information are impaired. PWCFS may have difficulty finding words and/or using words and numbers; they may have problems with altered spacial perceptions and abstract reasoning.

Cognitive dysfunction calls for adaptation, especially to perform tasks that must be done. When faced with college entrance examinations, for example, Trish applied for untimed Scholastic Achievement Testing. This would work toward alleviating the

## What Nurses Know...

*The percentage of CFS patients who recover is unknown, but there is some evidence to indicate that the sooner a person is treated, the better the chance of improvement. This means early diagnosis and treatment are important.*

stress of trying to respond to questions within a limited time. During high school, she met with some teachers who would accommodate her special needs. Despite having an individualized education plan, a special educational plan developed by the school's special education team, her parents, and herself to meet her academic goals and the means to achieve them, Trish did not always find teachers willing to follow the plan.

Cognitive dysfunction is a distressing CFS symptom. Some PWCFS experience symptom improvement when treated with the anticonvulsant, gabapentin (Neurontin). Scientists do not really know how this medication works but it appears to "even out" the nerve messages in the brain and helps the brain to respond to impulses at a steady rate.

For PWCFS who notice a slower response time, for example, to mental math, playing computer games may help "rewire" the brain pathways to work more efficiently. Computer games can help regain short-term memory and concentration.

Again, according to the Centers for Disease Control and Prevention (CDC):

*The severity of CFS varies from patient to patient, with some people able to maintain fairly active lives. For most symptomatic patients, however, CFS significantly limits work, school and family activities.*

While symptoms vary from person to person in number, type and severity, all CFS patients are functionally impaired to some degree. CDC studies show that CFS can be as disabling as multiple sclerosis, lupus, rheumatoid arthritis, heart disease, end-stage renal disease, chronic obstructive pulmonary disease (COPD) and similar chronic conditions.

CFS often follows a cyclical course, alternating between periods of illness and relative well-being. Some patients experience partial or complete remission of symptoms during the course of the illness, but symptoms often reoccur. This pattern of remission and relapse makes CFS especially hard for patients to manage. Patients who are in remission may be tempted to overdo activities when they're feeling better, which can actually cause a relapse.

The percentage of CFS patients who recover is unknown, but there is some evidence to indicate that the sooner a person is treated, the better the chance of improvement. This means early diagnosis and treatment are important.

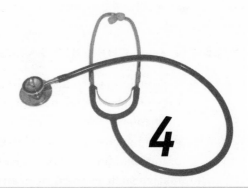

# Your Health Care Team

*For 24 years, I had the same caring physician who diagnosed me first with EBV, then CFS. He told me I'd be okay, that I needed to get more rest, and I'd get better. After three months, when I didn't get better, he became frustrated. He brushed me off to his young associate. Then he called me to cancel my next appointment with him. I now have a wonderful, knowledgeable physician, but my past experience has left me with trust issues when it comes to health care providers. People with CFS need a health care provider who believe and understand them as they direct their care.*   MARY

Mary's experience with her long-time health care provider (HCP) was unfortunate. It is difficult to find and keep an HCP who understands chronic fatigue syndrome (CFS). Especially when you are ill, you need someone who is knowledgeable and caring, and who validates how you feel.

You deserve someone who is qualified and will help you care for yourself. Ask friends or family members for referrals of HCPs they consult, or seek out a CFS organization or a CFS support group in your area that offers a referral service. Contact a local or national medical association that may furnish referral information such as The American Medical Association (http://www.ama-assn.org) or The American Board of Medical Specialties (http://www.abms.org).

Noted CFS researcher Lucinda Bateman, MD, who treats CFS patients, suggests calling your health plan to help you find a physician who can care for you. Find out more about the HCP's professional credentials and qualifications regarding treatment of CFS. According to Dr. Bateman, your primary practitioner need not be a CFS expert, but someone who is accessible, capable, and compassionate, and who can assess symptoms, provide a diagnostic workup to exclude other underlying conditions, and help with symptomatic care.

In your quest to find an HCP, call their office and request a telephone interview or make an appointment that will be an interview consultation. Find out if the HCP treats others with CFS, whether they accept your insurance, and research the hospital with which they are affiliated in case you need to be hospitalized. For example, "Are the HCPs affiliated with a small community hospital or a larger medical center with specialty departments, such as gastrointestinal, cardiac, or respiratory disease?"

The way the office staff treat you on the phone shows how they will treat you in the office. Pay attention to their tone of voice and whether they have a friendly, service attitude. If they leave you on hold, you may find the same treatment in the office.

Once in the office, notice how long you have to wait to be seen, whether the waiting room is comfortable for ill people, and how the HCP greets you. During the first contact, introduce yourself and present a summary or a mini-health history related to CFS. Notice whether the HCP listens to what you have to say.

When deciding on your HCPs, it is to your advantage to look for helpful qualities in them. In addition to being knowledgeable about CFS (or willing to learn about CFS), HCPs must believe you are ill, communicate effectively, listen to you, encourage you to ask questions, and answer your questions to the best of their ability or find resources that can provide answers. They must be willing to work with you as part of a team to develop a plan to manage your symptoms, set realistic goals for you to maintain or regain activities, and provide you with information regarding self-help and support groups for you and your family.

*If the health care provider you visit seems closed-minded to your illness, don't waist your energy. Go elsewhere. Ask a CFS support group for referrals. PWCFS need health care providers who understand.*   DIANA

## Team Members

There are a variety of health care professionals to choose for your health care team. Initially, you need to find someone to diagnose your illness and help manage your symptoms. To build your team, you may begin with one HCP as an overseer, perhaps a physician called a general practitioner or primary care physician, or an advanced practice nurse. In the United States, medicine is specialized, so a common approach to managing a multisystem illness like CFS is by using specialists who can be overseen by your choice of HCP who will refer you to these specialists.

Any decisions for referrals to specialists should be made jointly with your health care overseer. Typically, referrals are made based on CFS symptoms, their severity, and how long they have lasted. Severe symptoms, for example, warrant an immediate referral.

Getting referrals marks the beginning of the construction of your team with health care and allied health care professionals such as those listed below.

The **general practitioner, primary care physician** or **advanced practice nurse** (also called **nurse practitioner**) is the first contact person who may diagnose you or refer you to a specialist for tests to rule out other illnesses as part of the diagnostic process. These practitioners maintain your health records and could be called upon to verify your medical condition should you need disability insurance.

**Neurologists** specialize in treating diseases of the nervous system, including the brain, spinal cord, and the peripheral nervous system. They manage CFS symptoms such as migraine headache and pain.

**Rheumatologists** are doctors who specialize in processes that involve pain or movement disorders of joints and soft tissue, which may affect people with multisystem autoimmune diseases, fibromyalgia, and CFS.

**Pain management specialists** are doctors with specialized training in the diagnosis and management of pain.

**Gastroenterologists** are specialists who can assist you with digestive issues common to people with CFS (PWCFS), such as irritable bowel syndrome.

**Gynecologists** are physicians who specialize in women's health, treating diseases and illnesses that affect the female reproductive organs.

**Infectious disease specialists** are doctors of internal medicine (or, in some cases, pediatrics) who are qualified as experts in the diagnosis and treatment of infectious diseases such a measles, pneumonia, and hepatitis B. They also have additional training in immunology (how the body fights infection).

**Cardiologists** are specialists concerned with the functioning of the heart, blood vessels, and the circulation of the blood through the body.

**Nutritionists** are allied health care professionals who can help you establish a healthy eating plan and give you tips to prepare meals individualized to your body's needs.

**Occupational therapists** are allied health care professionals who can help you adapt to your environment and show you ways to make activities of daily living—such as housework and personal care—easier, and provide advice on useful aids or equipment.

**Physical therapists** are allied health care professionals who can provide you with advice on exercise, posture, and ways to relieve pain, as well as the use of treatments to maintain joint and muscle movement.

**Psychologists** are allied health care professionals who can teach you different ways of thinking about and coping with CFS.

**Rehabilitation counselors** are allied health care professionals who can help you with employment and retraining issues.

**Social workers** are allied health care professionals who can provide support and help with different aspects of your life that may be affected by your illness, such as your family life, income and housing, and other life problems.

Therapists who provide complementary and alternative medicine (CAM) therapies can be a valuable part of the health care team. CAM represents a group of diverse medical and health care systems and/or practices that are not generally considered part of conventional medicine.

Integrative therapists practice integrative medicine, that is, they combine conventional medicine and CAM treatments for which there is evidence of safety and effectiveness, for example, chiropractic and acupuncture. Once called alternative therapies, the new name reflects the concept that these treatments should be integrated into care rather than be considered an alternative to medical treatment. Acupuncture, for example, is the placement of small, thin needles at points along invisible meridians on the body, believed to correspond to the body's organs. This is believed to enable energy (called Qi in Chinese medicine) to flow more freely and enhance health. Research in China and in the

*To find a health care provider, do some homework. Check with your insurance carrier for providers covered by your plan or inquire about out-of-network coverage and charges. Check the provider's medical credentials and whether there have been any malpractice suits or disciplinary actions. There are several Web sites, such as RateMDs.com, where patients rate their doctors. Find out how other patients feel about a doctor whom you are considering.*

United States has shown that acupuncture, believed to enhance the immune system, can help lessen CFS symptoms and result in less pain, better sleep, and relaxation.

## Working With Your Team

It is important to build up a working relationship with your HCP and team by effectively communicating with them. This is hard work, especially when you are feeling ill and exhausted during your visits.

Communication begins with you. Encourage your HCPs to treat you as you need to be treated. During visits, show them that you respect their time, and they will respect you. Bring with you an organized checklist that prioritizes the most important issues you need to discuss. Perhaps your most pressing issue is the increased pain in your back that began a week ago. The HCP will discuss this with you, help you link the increased pain with a possible cause, and then suggest a treatment or refer you to a pain management specialist.

Your checklist should include a list of prescription and over-the-counter medications, including vitamins and supplements. This list will remind you to request needed refills giving the brand or generic name of the drug, the dose you take, and frequency with which you take it. For example, you might say,

*Patients should be encouraged to journal their symptoms. I designed a grid that we give out at our meeting. It is a check list, which makes it easy for a health care provider to see a month of symptoms on a single page. My doctor really likes it. With the 7.5 minutes allowed by insurance companies, there is not always time for lengthy explanations. It is too much information for the health care provider to absorb meaningfully at one time.* PAT

"I need a 90-day refill on Cymbalta, 20 mg, that I take twice a day." By knowing your medications, you show the HCP that you are a team player in your care.

Keeping a journal and a grid where you can check off problem symptoms is a helpful way to show HCPs how you have been feeling between visits. They offer concrete, visible answers to the HCPs' question, "How are you today?" With or without a journal or a grid, an example of a typical response to your HCP might be

"My lower back pain has gone up a bit. On a scale of 1 to 10, where 10 is the worst, I'm about a 6. This month I've been more tired. I think the change in the weather, all this rain, is affecting my pain level and my fatigue. I don't recall doing anything differently."

Waiting in the physician's office can further exhaust the CFS patient. When scheduling an appointment, explain this difficulty with the receptionist and try to schedule your next appointment when you can be seen first, typically the first visit of the day or immediately after lunch.

It is beneficial to bring a family member or patient advocate with you to help you express yourself when feeling ill or to record the HCP's recommendations. As time goes by, it is difficult and especially exhausting for PWCFS to remember their medical history. Keeping accurate records of what occurred during your visits and of your health history is part of your work to maintain your health. Again, this can be shared with a family member or patient advocate.

Although we are in an age of technology, as yet not all health care records are electronically stored and/or updated. The responsibility is on patients to keep their own, updated health records. Computer-savvy patients should enter and save their records in the computer. They can transfer their records to a memory stick, which they can bring to the computer-savvy HCP during visits. If the HCP does not have computer access in the office, patients can print out a copy of their records or part of their record to the HCP. Rather than overwhelm a new HCP, keep the record to a two-page minimum.

Ideally, your primary HCP can download a copy of your health record from your memory stick and be the keeper of your medical records from all other treating providers. Request each of your HCPs to send copies of their reports to the primary HCP who will update your medical record; otherwise, keep the record updated yourself or ask someone willing to do so. Remember to keep an updated copy on your flash drive for yourself.

The health information record can be organized according to headings such as those found on your own HCP's forms or those in the Medical History Table (see Table 4.1).

Begin your health information record with a paragraph that contains a list of past medical illnesses, serious injuries, and surgeries with their dates, for example, glaucoma both eyes, 1989; irritable bowel syndrome, 1990; hypertension, 2000; appendectomy, 2001; and fractured right elbow, 2002. Next, update your Medical History Table with current illnesses, symptoms, and treatments. Include a list of all HCPs with their contact information and the reason they are, or were, treating you.

To save your energy and everyone's time, request a copy of medical forms prior to an office visit, either via post or e-mail. Filling them out ahead of time, in a less stressful environment, assures accuracy.

Table 4.1    Medical History Table

| Current Diagnoses/ Date | Past Medical Tests/ Results/Dates | Family History | Treatment |
|---|---|---|---|
| CFS 2009 | Diagnosed by Dr. Smith, neurologist, based on symptoms (fatigue >6 months, new types of headache, swollen lymph nodes under arms, dizziness, sore throat, difficulty concentrating) | Cousin with CFS; aunt with fibromyalgia | Cymbalta one tablet (60 mg) morning and evening since 2010 |
| Sleep apnea 2008 | Sleep study 2008 | None | C-PAP (continuous positive airway pressure) machine at night |
| Heart palpitations 2007 | EKG, normal 2007 | Heart disease: father heart attack, died 2000 | None |
| Painful menstrual periods since 1990 | PAP smear, normal 2010 | Ovarian cancer: aunt died 2005 | Aleve two tablets as needed (440 mg) |
| Migraine headaches 2005 | MRI, normal 2005 | Father, uncle | Imitrex one tablet as needed (100 mg) |

As time goes by, it is difficult and especially exhausting for people with CFS (PWCFS) to remember their medical history. This Medical History Table was created by a PWCFS to help her remember and organize her medical information. PWCFS can use the questions on their health care providers' (HCPs) forms as a guide to creating their own Medical History Table. PWCFS should update the table frequently and bring it with them to HCPs' visits, especially any new HCP, to make sure HCPs' records are updated.

Once your team is in place and your symptom management is underway, your HCP should regularly review how you are faring. The time frame will depend on your needs and how you are managing with your symptoms and treatments. During a review, your primary HCP will assess any problems with medications or treatments, and assess your symptoms to see if they have changed significantly in any way. During this time, the primary HCP will help you determine whether you need a referral to a specialist, look at equipment you may need to help you with your daily activities, or help you seek benefits, such as disability insurance, to which you may be entitled.

Just as Mary's bad experience with her long-time HCP has left her with trust issues, researchers have found that fear and lack of trust and confidence in HCPs are barriers to using health care services. Patients with fatiguing illnesses often forego needed medical care because they tend to self-diagnose their symptoms such as muscle and joint pains, headache, or sleeping problems. As a consequence of self-diagnosis, they self-treat their symptoms with over-the-counter medications. This approach may lead to more serious health problems later.

Often, PWCFS see multiple specialists without the benefit of an HCP overseer; however, teaming up with your HCP will

## What Nurses Know...

Health care providers (HCPs) are stressed and overworked; however, it is their job to provide you with the care you deserve. Do your best to find HCPs who will work with you as part of a team. If you have a bad experience with one and it cannot be remedied, move on. When it comes to your health, it is your life that is on the line.

improve the care you receive. It is important to learn how to talk to your HCP, and ask questions about your medical issues, treatment, and drugs. Take time to educate those HCPs who do not understand CFS. Strive to work together to manage your symptoms and better your quality of life.

## A Word About Caregivers

Caregivers are called to the special work of helping PWCFS maintain a good quality of life. Their work varies with the symptoms and the intensity of symptoms that PWCFS experience. Whether the caregiver is a spouse, a parent, sibling, or friend, day to day they rise to the challenge of thinking about the other person, making sure they are all right.

Caregivers' support is invaluable. Many PWCFS are very ill and need much assistance. Although caregivers generously provide care, they need to know about CFS and how it has affected—and can in the future affect—the person they care for. Some effects of CFS of which caregivers must be aware include the following:

- The once active PWCFS must now spend time away from their work or school and rely on others for help, which can induce feelings of anger, sadness, or guilt.
- Fatigue or malaise may cause PWCFS to avoid making advance plans, cancel planned activities, and become socially withdrawn.
- Because they typically do not look ill, friends, family, and some HCPs may think they are making up their illness. The unkind reactions of some may lead to their lack of confidence or self-esteem.
- Well-meaning friends or uninformed HCPs may encourage PWCFS to do more than they are able, which can trigger a relapse or postexertional malaise. Instead, PWCFS need to be encouraged to pace themselves.

- CFS can take a significant toll on families, resulting in spouses unable to cope and financial difficulties from lack of employment.

The top priority for caregivers is to offer physical and emotional support. Caregivers should keep an open line of communication with PWCFS by being nonjudgmental toward both them and the professionals with whom they must collaborate. Because PWCFS often experience disbelief that "they are still ill" or have a "real" illness, they need validation. Confirm your belief in them and their illness. If an HCP shows doubt, offer to help them find a supportive HCP. Regarding personal communication, use the following as a guide to action:

- Ask PWCFS what they need and how you can help. Listen to them rather than providing suggestions on how to "fix" things.
- Offer support and be understanding when they cancel plans due to illness or fatigue.
- Offer positive responses such as, "I'm sorry you're feeling so bad" or "You're handling things so well," or "I know this is difficult for you."
- Avoid comments such as, "You can beat this thing, if you try hard." Avoid negative comparisons such as, "You walked for a longer time yesterday" or "You used to have such energy."

When PWCFS are too ill to act for themselves, caregivers become advocates. They facilitate communication between HCPs. They may drive them to and attend medical appointments, helping PWCFS report their most pressing problems, ask appropriate questions, and take notes about the medical recommendations.

For PWCFS who need help with daily living activities, caregivers can make note of what activities they have difficulty completing, such as getting dressed or balancing the check-book. Offer specific help, for example, by laying out clothing, helping organize bills, or computing bank balances. Suggest that PWCFS always keep needed items, such as keys, in a specific place where they can easily be found. Suggest that they write down directions or have someone else do it for them.

It is important for caregivers to educate themselves about CFS and how to be good caregivers, and also to take care of themselves at the same time. They should realize their limitations, take "time off" when possible, and seek support for themselves from local CFS organizations, friends, and HCPs. Caregivers can sometimes feel angry or guilty and may need to talk with a friend or another support person. There are Internet discussion groups for caregivers of PWCFS and other chronic illnesses such as CFS-Care. Here, topics discussed include emotional support, communication, research, diagnosis and treatment, related illnesses, support mechanisms, community, and humor.

By looking into support for themselves, caregivers are better able to support PWCFS. Perhaps the answer lies in creating

## What Nurses Know . . .

Caring for someone else can be very stressful. Caregivers must take care of themselves in order to take care of the other person. The following are some important tips for caregivers:

- Maintain your health
- Accept help from others
- Make time for yourself
- Stay connected with others
- Speak to a counselor

a support network, creating a list of family, friends, neighbors, and coworkers who can help with certain aspects of care. Calling on others can decrease the risk of caregiver burnout and form a community of care for PWCFS.

Caregivers should set reasonable expectations for the care they are able to offer, enjoy their own lives, friends, and activities, and give themselves credit for the assistance they provide.

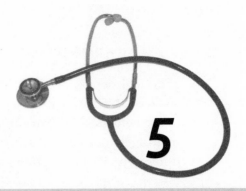

# Save Energy, Keep up With Living, Prevent Postexertional Malaise

*I don't know what it means to save up [my] energy. I don't have energy to save. It's not something I can conceive of. I plan one goal, something fairly simple to do around the house each day, and even if I don't get to do it, it helps to have something to look forward to.* MARYANNE

People are individuals who learn to cope with chronic illness in their own way. When it comes to expending energy, it is well to remember that no blanket advice fits all people with chronic fatigue syndrome (PWCFS). PWCFS are a diverse group who vary with age, severity of illness, different stages of chronic fatigue syndrome (CFS), existence of overlapping medical conditions, weight, pre-illness state of body conditioning, and amount of deconditioning due to illness. These factors impact how a person with CFS responds to activity.

Symptoms of CFS vary from person to person and day to day, making it more (or less) difficult to function. It helps to hear how others with CFS deal with symptoms, keep up with living, try to prevent relapses, and try to "save" energy. Although MaryAnne cannot imagine what it is like to save up energy, she copes with her lack of energy by setting small goals to achieve daily.

Even on "good" days, PWCFS benefit from not overextending themselves. Even on "good" days, it is helpful to sit whenever possible rather than stand, take rest breaks, and pace yourself. Shopping trips can be cut down to more manageable portions of time or done via computer. Make a list of priorities for the day and aim to do what it is that you truly love to do.

For PWCFS who are in pain and experience fatigue, low energy, and brain fog, it is difficult to get going. Your health care provider (HCP) may suggest taking antidepressant medications that address the imbalance of the brain chemicals (neurotransmitters) serotonin, norepinephrine, or dopamine to address these symptoms that may be related to this imbalance.

*Find out what makes you feel good inside, something that gets you through the day when you can't do what you want to do. Know what you like and what makes you feel good without any stress or pain, or what will make it worse. Accept that you can't do what you wanted to, and tell yourself, "That will be for another day."* MARYANNE

## Exercise

PWCFS have a broad range of ability when it comes to activity. Although some can gradually increase their strength and aerobic capacity and even recover to a higher level of function, others who attempt to increase activity experience relapse of symptoms either immediately or within a few weeks. Fear of relapse or postexertional malaise (PEM) can lead to lack of motivation to be active.

Lack of motivation and the resulting lack of physical activity bring with them a lack of physical conditioning. This creates a cycle of tiredness where people too tired to exercise become physically unfit, making them more susceptible to tiredness. Although lying down may make you feel better, being physically inactive can make you stiff and sore, and result in deconditioning.

Rather than aiming for aerobic exercise, PWCFS need to redefine exercise as the activity they can carry out according to their ability. The Centers for Disease Control and Prevention recommends that PWCFS work with their health care professionals to create an individualized exercise program that focuses on interval activity or graded exercise. The goal is to balance rest and activity to avoid both deconditioning from lack of activity and flare-ups of illness due to overexertion. A realistic goal for severely ill patients is to focus on improving flexibility and minimizing the impact of deconditioning in order to increase function enough to manage basic activities.

Nationally recognized CFS consultant and Director of the Hunter-Hopkins Center, P.A., Medical Consultations, in Charlotte, NC, Charles Lapp, MD, advises his CFS patients (who can be active) to be active, to set limits on their activity, and to avoid the tendency to push 'n' crash or to not do anything at all for fear of triggering symptoms. He suggests that they try to accomplish things in small steps, followed by 10-to-30-minute rest periods two to three times during the day.

According to Dr. Lapp, activity plans must be highly individualized, based on personal tolerances and abilities. PWCFS should begin and increase slowly with an activity-to-rest ratio of 1:3; for example, after exercising for 30 seconds, the person would rest for 90 seconds. The PWCFS must respect the threshold and not increase length of time when the exercise is not well tolerated, and must limit the time of any sustained action initially to 30-60 seconds and the entire activity to 5 minutes. Five minutes, three times a day is better tolerated than a 15-minute block of activity, yet the results in conditioning are equivalent.

PWCFS should consult their HCPs before adopting an exercise program. One example of a CFS activity program that Dr. Lapp recommends consists initially of exercises that help with activities of daily living and moves on to strengthening and conditioning exercises, for example, hand stretches, sitting and standing, picking up and grasping objects, light stretching, and strengthening exercises using only the body's weight as resistance. When these are mastered and well-tolerated, stretch bands and light weights may be added, followed by aerobic activities like walking, biking, or pool therapy. Everything is individualized.

When explaining the concept of energy conservation, Dr. Lapp uses the example of energy dollars (EDs). Every activity has an energy cost. The goal is to have some EDs left at the end of each day, for example, if you begin with 10 EDs, aim to have 2 EDs left. If you spend more EDs than you have, you have to make them up the next day.

There are ways to monitor activity so that PWCFS who are able to be active do not overdo or underdo it. Dr. Lapp advises able patients to take from 1,000 to 5,000 steps each day as measured by a pedometer. They should stay within the aerobic threshold (AT)—the heart rate during exercise needed to have a training effect. This is a heart rate halfway between the resting heart rate and the maximum heart rate (determined by the HCP). Patients can limit the time they spend or the heart rate so as not to exceed the AT (thus trying to avoid a flare up of symptoms). After exercise, patients should ask themselves how they feel afterward as well as the next day.

Activity must be approached with caution and a sense of balance. Rather than fearing and not engaging in any activity, PWCFS must attempt what they can, know their limitations, and pace themselves to avoid aftereffects.

## Conserving Energy

Conserving energy can be as simple as careful body positioning. Good posture, for example, lessens unnecessary muscle tension that drains energy. Whether sitting or standing, be mindful to have good posture where you hold your head and back straight with your arms relaxed at the shoulders. This balances the weight of your head and limbs on the bony framework so that the force of gravity helps keep joint position. The further you move from this position, the more energy is required of your muscles to pull against gravity to maintain your position.

## Pacing Yourself

Executive director and founder of the Chronic Fatigue and Immune Dysfunction Syndrome and Fibromyalgia Self-Help Program, Bruce Campbell, PhD, advocates pacing oneself to gain control over CFS symptoms. After a four-year bout with

## *What Nurses Know...*

### CORRECT ENERGY-DRAINING POSITIONS

- *To avoid energy-draining positions, do not shrug your shoulders or hunch over when sitting at a desk.*
- *Keep your head straight up rather than in a forward position when reading or at the computer.*
- *Use a high stool with back support.*
- *Make it a point to be aware of your body's position.*
- *Note the positions that caused energy drain and think of ways to correct the problem.*

CFS, Dr. Campbell says he has recovered ninety percent and recommends pacing oneself as a way of living with CFS.

According to Dr. Campbell, every type of activity from standing, talking, driving, or using a computer has its own limit. Pacing strategies include setting activity limits, reducing activity levels, taking daily planned rests regardless of how the person is feeling, switching among tasks, and keeping detailed records. It also includes making mental adjustments based on the acceptance that life has changed.

When it comes to exerting energy, patience is important because doing too much at once and exceeding your limits results in payback. Symptoms return, and can do so with a vengeance. Your limit is called your threshold. When you go beyond it, you can trigger PEM, a defining feature of CFS whose cause is unknown. PEM varies from escalation of widespread pain, to exhaustion requiring a recovery day in bed, to serious relapse of the entire CFS symptom complex: the cognitive dysfunction, flu-like achiness, fatigue, low-grade fevers, lymph node tenderness, and disturbed sleep patterns that can last weeks or months. PEM is out of proportion to the event that triggered it.

Pacing can help PWCFS avoid both over- and under-exertion, and may reduce the frequency and severity of PEM. Patients can choose from a wide variety of techniques and practices to create their own customized pacing program. CFS researcher Leonard Jason, PhD, advises CFS patients (who have little stamina and endurance) not to "push their energy envelope"; that is, they should pace their activity according to their available energy resources. Dr. Jason says that maintaining expended energy levels consistent with available energy levels may reduce the frequency and severity of symptoms. In a study of CFS patients, Dr. Jason found that participants in his study who expended energy beyond their level of perceived energy would have more severe fatigue and symptoms and lower levels of physical and mental functioning.

How do PWCFS find out about their own energy envelopes? Dr. Campbell suggests making a list of activities that you do daily and can do, along with the time period in which you can do them without bringing on CFS symptoms. For example, if you walk for 15 minutes each day, write that down along with how your body reacts to this activity. By keeping this activity journal, you can find activities that need adjustment, perhaps an increase or decrease in the amount of time or change of location. Knowing what you can and cannot do can help improve your quality of life.

*Keeping a diary helped me see patterns of my illness and head off certain flare-ups.* STEVE

## Avoiding PEM

To try to avoid PEM, get an overall picture of how you spend your EDs. Energy means more than physical activities. In your assessment, include mental activities such as reading, working on the computer, and concentrating on something. Think of social activities like talking on the phone or the time you have been with others. Consider your emotions, which can run the gamut from frustration, anxiety, and stress, to happiness.

Special events are stressors that subtract from your EDs. These include vacations, holiday celebrations, having dinner guests, or going out of the house for various appointments, and call for strategic planning to avoid PEM. These activities, as well as feeling pressured by others or yourself to be more active, can be a cause for PEM or a relapse.

PWCFS can use strategies to meet the challenge of special events. Dr. Campbell suggests that PWCFS take extra rest before an event and extra rest afterward. If participating in a long activity, for example, sitting in class for 2 hours, take a stretch or bathroom break. Before the event, make a detailed plan to include alternate activities you can do if your energy level is being depleted. For example, choose the parts of a family outing that you can participate in and enjoy. Discuss your plans with others involved in the event so they understand what to expect from you. Being upfront with others regarding what you will participate in may reduce their trying to encourage your full participation.

PWCFS must define their limits, simplify their tasks at hand, substitute or eliminate demanding tasks with less demanding ones, and delegate chores. If it is a "good" day for company to come, for example, keep it simple. Enlist family to help you prepare food for the guests and clean up afterward. Know your time limit for entertaining and make this clear to your guests beforehand. Do not be tempted to extend the time because you will pay for it later.

It is difficult to accept that you are not the same as you were before CFS. Rather than make this comparison, listen to your body's signals and remind yourself that you are resting so that you can return to finish the task at hand. Dr. Campbell suggests changing the negative way of thinking, "I'm weak if I need to rest," to "If I rest, I'll have quality time with my husband and grandchildren."

PEM is unpredictable. Researchers have not yet found the cause or treatment; however, PWCFS can use strategies to try to minimize it. Pacing is one way that PWCFS can help themselves. Pacing is not a cure for PEM or for CFS. While some patients may be able to be active, other patients may not; however, pacing, and being able to prevent PEM to some degree, gives CFS patients some power over the illness. If a patient can predict the consequences of an activity, that patient is empowered to make informed choices.

*I found myself in bed full time because of CFS/ME. I was just lying there doing nothing and not improving. Then, through some fortunate events, I discovered a different approach, one that has shown me a way to reduce my symptoms and to gain a sense of control. Even though I am still quite limited, I now have a sense of purpose and hope for the first time in years.*   GERALDINE

## For the Bedbound

As Geraldine found out, pacing and the right mindset can be valuable for bedbound people living with CFS. After a prolonged period of bed rest, her HCP referred Geraldine to an occupational therapist who taught her pacing as a new way to live with CFS.

First Geraldine needed to find out her baseline, an amount of activity that did not intensify her symptoms and that could be sustained on both good and bad days. She determined her baselines by keeping a two-week diary of each activity every hour and then recorded her fatigue level afterward. When she saw that she could actually do less than she thought, she realized that she had to very slowly increase her activity level, sometimes only a minute at a time.

Geraldine also categorized her activities as high, medium, and low energy and divided them into a series of steps. For her, high energy activities included showering and bathing, holding conversations, using the telephone, and watching television. Medium-level activities included cooking and laundry. Low-energy activities included resting quietly, using the laptop in bed, and listening to the radio through headphones.

To make activities more manageable, Geraldine divided them into small parts. For example, if she needed to make a phone call, she would write down exactly what she needed to say, and practice it. She would anticipate the reply and determine what she would say in response, and practice that. If she had to cook a meal, she would divide it into stages. In the morning, she would prepare the veggies and meat. In the afternoon, she would set the table, and do the actual cooking in the evening.

Pacing brings structure to the life of people living with CFS by providing achievable goals. When written down in a journal and checked off as achieved, these goals give patients a sense of control and purpose in life.

> *Life [with CFS] is a balancing act. Each day is renewed, and you figure out what you can and cannot, should or should not, do. I try not to push myself and do more than is good for me, but on some [rare] days, I choose to push myself to the limits. I'm not happy about feeling sicker later, but I know I'm doing it [that day] for a good reason. Trying to keep your mental and emotional being filled, without damaging the physical, is a very hard balance.* MARYANNE

Regardless of where you are with your CFS symptoms, life on a regular schedule, balanced with rest, is helpful. As part of his recuperative strategy, Dr. Campbell found that sticking to a daily schedule stabilized his life. Dr. Campbell set aside planned 15-minute rest periods where he would lie down in a quiet room, eyes closed, in the morning and in the afternoon, to recharge his batteries. He found that using mental relaxation techniques during these rest periods deepened the restorative power of his rest. This is a preemptive type of rest that is nurturing and can lead to having more energy with lower symptom levels. They are a useful part of pacing, which helps patients gain a sense of control over their illness by living according to a plan rather than in response to symptoms.

> *One woman with CFS told me she was supposed to go out to lunch with friends, but cancelled several times. She is an early riser and was too tired by lunchtime to go out. I suggested she set aside an hour or so beforehand to lie down*

*and rest. She said she was going to try this—or perhaps meet for breakfast.*    PAT

## Balance Is Key

Balancing your life with rest and activity makes for a more stress-free lifestyle. It also calls for making changes to your current one. Think about what you would change to nurture yourself. Consider the following supports that can help you do so.

- Get a handicap sticker for your car to save steps walking to your destination.
- Do not make too many commitments. Learn how to say no and to delegate tasks.
- Consider adapting your daily living activities to your needs. For example, take a bath instead of a shower to save energy and limit the possibility of getting dizzy and falling. If you must shower, do so at night to help you sleep.
- Whenever possible, sit instead of standing, for example, when preparing food or combing your hair.
- Keep a metal shopping cart or small hand truck in your car to avoid having to carry groceries or other items.
- Work on your sense of humor by watching comedies and reading jokes and positive books to distract you from daily stress.
- Make lists of things to do that make you feel happy. Aim to do one a day.
- Find support from an in-person or online support group, or a phone or e-mail buddy.
- Try to maintain friendships—even when homebound. Visit by phone.

Keep your expectations realistic. Aim to gradually increase what you can manage over time. You may take two steps forward and two or more backward, but the idea is to keep forging ahead.

## A Word About Nutrition

Adequate nutrition is key to good health. There is no standard "CFS" diet. Selecting proper foods and avoiding others, as well as preparing food to eat, are challenging for PWCFS. For example, some PWCFS who have overlapping conditions that affect digestion and elimination, such as irritable bowel syndrome, face the challenge of finding nutritious food that does not cause intestinal pain, diarrhea, heartburn, or gas. The process is more complicated if you can tolerate a certain food one day, but have a negative reaction the next time you eat it. Experiment if the reaction is not a serious one. Perhaps you can tolerate that food only occasionally. Listen to your body.

Many people living with CFS experience intolerance of alcohol, caffeine, and sweeteners (such as sugar, corn syrup, fructose, aspartame, and saccharin), food additives (such as monosodium glutamate, preservatives, artificial colors, and artificial flavors), and tobacco. Cutting down or eliminating these substances may reduce symptoms and mood swings, and may improve sleep.

Consider whether your food reactions may be caused by celiac disease, a sensitivity to wheat products, or lactose intolerance to milk products. See an HCP who will help determine if this is the cause of your food reactions and provide a diet that you need to follow.

Other PWCFS have sensitivities or allergies to foods that may make them feel ill with headaches, muscle pain, or fatigue. Although some PWCFS may be allergic to wheat, eggs, corn, or dairy products, others are not. It is important to identify foods that trigger negative reactions by eliminating them one at a time from your diet for several days. Make note of what you have eliminated and whether the symptom subsided during that time.

Then try eating that food again to see if the negative symptoms return.

PWCFS may have a lack of appetite when symptoms flare up. Many PWCFS have nutritional deficiencies, but it is difficult to determine if this is the cause or a result of the disease. Typically, PWCFS are low in B vitamins, magnesium, vitamin D, and many other nutrients. Deficiencies in vitamins and minerals can lead to health problems that can mimic symptoms of CFS. Low vitamin D, for example, can mimic a syndrome similar to CFS with muscle pain and weakness. Low vitamin B12 with fibromyalgia creates a worsened chronic pain syndrome and peripheral neuropathy (numbness and/or pain in the hands and feet).

They may be too tired to use their energy to prepare meals. At this time, friends or family members may be able to share some of the meal preparation. If possible, preparing meals in advance; freezing them for these "down" times can be helpful. A friend or family member can be called on to defrost the meal and ensure that you will be eating well.

On days when you are feeling well enough, try to cook more than what is necessary and package and freeze portions that can be defrosted and cooked when you are not feeling up to it. Commercially used frozen foods could be used, although

## What Nurses Know...

*If cooking for 20 minutes causes too much pain or fatigue, it is too much for you. Make a note of when you began and stopped cooking. Include how much pain and fatigue you felt. Compare this with how you felt on another day when you did the same amount of cooking but stopped to rest for a break after 10 minutes.*

because of the high sodium content, it is not recommended to rely on them.

Dealing with CFS really means a lifestyle change. Learn to slow down and pace yourself. Individualize an exercise routine that helps rather than exacerbates your fatigue—and always aim to reduce stress.

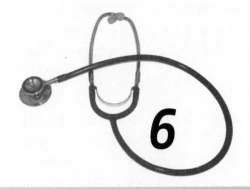

# Feelings, Mood Swings, and Depression

*It's so upsetting not to be able to function day, after day, after day. I know I don't want to feel sorry for myself or feel down about it. This realization is key because my attitude is the one thing I have control over and can work on. This makes a big difference in my life. I won't say I always win, but most of the time I do pretty well with it. It's a daily battle.* MARYANNE

## Empowerment: Sick and Tired of Being Sick and Tired

MaryAnne, a mother with three grandchildren, has been ill for more than twenty years and was diagnosed with chronic fatigue syndrome (CFS)/fibromyalgia about five years ago. "The diagnosis is vague, like the symptoms," says MaryAnne. "The doctors don't agree. One says I have chronic Epstein–Barr virus, another lupus, and another that it's all psychological."

"I feel like a hypochondriac or a broken record because I've got these symptoms and the illness is hard to diagnose and treat. After testing for everything else, CFS is the diagnosis that has stayed [with me]."

Imagine having the achy tiredness of the flu, but the feeling never subsides. You might have a brief reprieve, but no matter what you do, the symptoms return, and you're back to square one. That is the cycle of CFS symptoms. It is no wonder that people with CFS (PWCFS) are sick and tired of being sick and tired. As with all chronic illnesses, CFS symptoms, new lifestyle restrictions, social isolation caused from the fatigue, or the lack of being diagnosed can lead to feelings of depression that may express itself as sadness, worthlessness, or guilt.

It is incorrect to assume that CFS is a form of depression or that all people living with CFS have depression. However, it is not uncommon to see both depression and CFS in the same person.

Depression is a common but serious illness where the people affected experience a lasting sadness that interferes with their quality of life. People with depression have a sense of hopelessness, helplessness, and feelings of excessive guilt and self-criticism. These are not *primary* symptoms expressed by PWCFS. Unlike PWCFS, people with depression have lost almost all interest in what they used to enjoy. They often have low self-esteem, unreasonable guilt, and feelings of hopelessness. Typically, PWCFS want to be interested in what they used to enjoy, but are just too tired.

CFS and depression are two distinct disorders. Some symptoms of depression are similar to CFS, such as change in weight, fatigue and low energy, and difficulty concentrating and making decisions. People with depression do not generally experience most of the physical and neurologic deficits seen in

## What Nurses Know...

*People living with CFS want to do things and be active, but they can't. People with depression have lost the desire to do things.*

PWCFS, which can include sore throat, tender and/or swollen lymph nodes, unusual headaches, muscle and joint pain, muscle twitching and fatigue, nausea, irritable bowel syndrome, unusual sensitivities to medications, postexertional malaise (PEM), visual and auditory disturbances, speech and language deficits, altered spatial perception, clumsiness and coordination problems, disequilibrium, autonomic disturbances such as neurally mediated hypotension, thermoregulation, and others.

*What works best for me is keeping my attitude positive no matter what each day brings. I make sure I do enough socially, which is very hard because I want to go out, but [at the same time] I don't want to do anything [because of the fatigue from CFS]. I phone friends a lot and I watch TV, which makes me feel related.*   MARYANNE

## Symptoms Distinguish CFS From Depression

After exercise, people with depression generally feel better. Studies show that exercise boosts serotonin, the pleasure hormone in the brain, making people feel better. PWCFS have exercise intolerance and can experience PEM, a period of intense exhaustion, and other CFS symptoms that last for more than 24 hours. PEM is a hallmark of CFS. Researchers are studying the muscles of PWCFS who have PEM triggered by exercise.

They have found that it takes longer for the muscles of PWCFS to return to their normal pre-exercise state. These detectable differences show up in the blood and are being studied as possible markers to diagnose CFS.

*Some days I choose to push myself to the limits, but I pay for it. I'm not happy about feeling sicker afterward, but I know I chose to push myself for a reason. I can't do that often.* MARYANNE

The classic CFS symptoms, such as joint and muscle pain, severe headaches, recurrent sore throats and upper respiratory infections, tender lymph nodes, and rapid heart beat are not common to people with depression. People living with CFS may have poor immunity and have recurrent infections that people with depression do not. As with others who have chronic debilitating illnesses, some PWCFS may develop depression as a reaction to the impairments caused by the symptoms and their reduced quality of life. Depression can also be a side effect of, or reaction to, medications.

Sleep can be a distinguishing factor between CFS and depression. Some people with depression may often have insomnia while those with CFS usually do not. Others who have CFS or depression may either sleep more than usual or may experience non-restful sleep; however, the type of sleep disturbances that often accompany CFS are not common in people with depression. During sleep, the brains of PWCFS generate "awake" sleep signals when they should be in deep, restorative sleep. This prevents their bodies from repairing and healing. No matter how long they sleep, PWCFS do not feel refreshed when they wake up. According to the health care provider who diagnosed my daughter with CFS, Trisha responded with a classic answer to "How do you feel in the morning when you wake up?" Trisha answered, "I feel like I've been hit by a truck."

# Sleep

Even healthy people feel "down" when their sleep is disrupted or decreased. Research has shown that when people's sleep is interrupted or when they have lost sleep, their mood is affected and they have a decrease in cognitive and physical performance and experience muscle discomfort and sensitivity to pain. Imagine having disrupted or decreased sleep, night after night. Nearly all PWCFS have problems getting restorative, refreshing sleep, which can reinforce many symptoms of CFS. Getting a restful night's sleep is a tremendous hurdle that is difficult to overcome, but practical actions can make sleep possible.

Whether or not to take medications for sleep is a serious decision because many medications have side effects. There are no perfect medications for sleep, and most have side effects. It is important to weigh those side effects with whether the medication helps you to get to sleep and provides a better quality of sleep. As a person with CFS, you must be aware that you are more sensitive to medication. Health care providers who recommend medications usually encourage PWCFS to start with a lower dose than they would prescribe for people who do not have CFS. They may suggest using a lower dose of an antihistamine such as Benadryl. They may suggest that patients keep a record of how they respond to the medication to see if it is effective and to adjust the dose to the patient's needs.

Some of the medications that have been recommended as possible sleep aids are not really considered sleeping medications, but when used for sleep can be taken regularly to keep you asleep or work toward keeping you asleep. These include various prescription antidepressants, pain medications that may cause drowsiness and sleep, and over-the-counter medications such as melatonin, a natural hormone normally produced in our bodies. Melatonin is used primarily to regulate the body's natural clock and address insomnia. Although melatonin is generally considered safe, it may cause daytime sleepiness. Those who drive should do so with caution. When any medication is considered, it is important for people to consult with their health care providers to avoid drug interactions and harmful side effects. A drug that might work for one person may not work for another, or may cause side effects in one but not the other.

No studies have examined the effectiveness of Ambien in CFS, but anecdotal evidence would suggest it is not as effective with PWCFS as other sleep medications.

The challenge with treating sleep problems in PWCFS is that they can be grouped into two categories: those who have non-restorative sleep from the lack of deep (rapid eye movement) sleep (the majority), and those who have or develop sleep apnea over time where they fall into deeper sleep with a disordered breathing pattern that leads to a decrease in oxygen. A sleep expert can perform a sleep study test to determine if PWCFS have sleep apnea, or PWCFS can be given a pulse oximeter (that looks like a small clamp) to wear on their finger while they are sleeping at night to determine whether they have sleep apnea. A sleep expert can listen to the whole sleep story and help determine treatment.

## Sleep Hygiene

Getting into a sleep routine with good sleep hygiene can be helpful. Noted researcher, Dr. Richard Podell, suggests the following principles of sleep hygiene.

- Discuss whether medicines, for example, decongestants, diet pills, or stimulating antidepressants—and also evening caffeine or alcohol—might be disrupting sleep.
- Keep sleep schedules regular. Shifting sleep time disrupts sleep. Create a habit pattern of staging down activities throughout the evening. This helps condition your body to be able to sleep. Consider turning the TV off early. Try music or dull reading.
- Keep the bedroom dark and quiet and the mattress comfortable. Leave marital conflicts outside.

- Use the bed only for sleep or sex.
- Clear your mind of the past days' events and the next days' worries. Write down your regrets and plans, then lock them in a drawer so you can go back to them the next day.
- Do not exercise just before bedtime.
- Consider a hot bath in the early evening. Heat initially prompts alertness; drowsiness then follows as your body temperature drops.
- Take a modest carbohydrate snack or warm milk before sleep. This promotes drowsiness for some.
- Use relaxation tapes, imagery, slow diaphragmatic breathing, or meditation.
- Use ear plugs to avoid too much noise and eye shades to avoid too much light.
- Use white noise, a fan, or calm music to soothe out and block unwanted sounds.

## Determining Depression

Although any illness can trigger feelings of depression, people with a chronic illness such as CFS are at greater risk of being depressed. People with a chronic illness find it more difficult to deal with everyday stress. They find it harder to perform their everyday tasks at home and at work and may begin to think of themselves as helpless or hopeless. They may feel out of control and become depressed. When caused by chronic illness,

## What Nurses Know...

*Tossing and turning, trying to get to sleep is frustrating. Sleep techniques can help, but what is good for one may not be helpful for another person with CFS. Trial and error is a good method to find what is right for you.*

depression can make the pain and fatigue worse. This sets up a vicious cycle, as the person who feels worse begins to seek isolation which, in turn, makes the depression worse.

To determine whether a person with CFS has depression, health care providers can administer brief psychiatric screening tools such as the Beck Depression Inventory or the Patient Health Questionnaire nine-item depression scale. Results of these screening tools can point to a possible underlying depression or other psychological disorder. The health care provider can then refer the person to a mental health professional.

Early diagnosis of depression is important so that treatment can begin as soon as possible. If symptoms of depression are the result of medications, these can be changed or adjusted to help relieve the symptoms. Physicians and psychiatrists work with people with depression to find the medication and treatment that is most helpful for them.

> *Getting up in [the] morning is always hard. I'm a morning person, but it's hard to get going. Things get a little better as the day goes on, so in the morning I tell myself that it'll get better. It helps to keep positive.* MARYANNE

## Cognitive–Behavioral Therapy

Cognitive-behavioral therapy (CBT) is an individualized psychological therapy provided by specially trained health care providers such as psychologists, nurses, or physical or occupational therapists that may be considered as part of the management of chronic illnesses such as depression and CFS. Rather than the traditional therapy that dwells on the past, CBT focuses on current issues and symptoms. During CBT, people examine their beliefs, concerns, and coping behaviors, and modify them to develop constructive coping strategies.

CBT is a therapy, not a cure. During this therapy, physical activity is slowly introduced, based on an individual's activity tolerance, and must be carefully monitored so as not to cause PEM or a relapse. Although CBT is considered controversial by many in the patient advocacy community, it can help some patients and families to understand the illness and how to live with it. Although CBT is an effective part of the management of chronic diseases such as cancer, rehabilitation of orthopedic injuries, and depressive disorders, according to the Centers for Disease Control and Prevention, the utility of CBT for CFS is in its formative stages and much needs to be learned before the full extent or limits of its usefulness are known.

The CFIDS Association of America, committed to advancing research that leads to the early detection, objective diagnosis, and effective treatment of CFS, alerts PWCFS that headlines regarding studies about CBT and graded exercise can be misleading, especially those that tout treatments as leading to a cure. According to the CFIDS Association of America president, Kim McCleary, these headlines contribute to dismissive attitudes about CFS and undermine the understanding of its severe and life-altering impact. They vastly oversimplify the individual patient's ability to recover his or her health.

Rather than attempt more aggressive regimens than their bodies can withstand, PWCFS need to listen to their bodies, and work with health care professionals who recommend and deliver individualized care that will take PEM into account.

As McCleary says,

*Structured programs that seek to expand function and reduce symptoms may provide modest benefits when added to standard medical care, but they do not offer complete resolution of symptoms or cure. According to the effects seen in younger people, less severely ill, and more recently ill, these groups may benefit more, but there are risks to these therapies, especially when used outside the standardized setting of research studies.*

*What Nurses Know...*

When left untreated, symptoms of depression can actually make other symptoms worse; for example, anxiety causes stress. Stress contributes to pain, fatigue, and inability to sleep.

Living with CFS is a balancing act. Each day you have to figure out what you can, should, or shouldn't do. You have to try to keep your "mental and emotional being" filled without damaging your physical being. It's a very hard balance.  MARYANNE

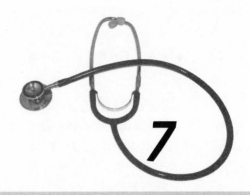

7

# Medical Treatments for Chronic Fatigue Syndrome

*If a pharmacist looks at an inventory of all the medications I've tried, they might assume I've been diagnosed with any or all of: depression, anxiety, bipolar mania, schizophrenia, insomnia, arthritis, asthma, chronic sinusitis, and chronic rhinitis. They also may wonder whether or not I'll end up in a drug rehab center, given the extensive list of narcotic pain killers and narcotic cough medications (from the consistently recurring bronchitis and pneumonia resulting from the sinusitis-induced postnasal drip), in addition to the long list of potentially addictive wake-promoting medications and the potentially addictive sleep-promoting agents I take to counter the wake-promoting drugs (and hopefully help obtain the restorative sleep from which CFS deprives me).*

*From a patient's perspective, the hardest part of treating CFS is maintaining the emotional strength to endure the years spent living as a medical "guinea pig." It's a process that takes years, and truthfully never stops. Mom and I spent the first few years looking for answers, reasons, and cures. When we came to the realization that the "answer" meant accepting that there is no answer, no reason, and no cure, it took me years to grieve. I know my parents grieved too, but they found the strength to hide that from me. I remember thinking that their consistently positive attitude was naively optimistic, but now that I'm older I understand why they did it, and admire that they found the courage to do so. Through their fortitude, I found the strength to move forward and resolve to take each day and each symptom one step at a time. I can still hear Mom and Dad saying, "Trisha, how do you eat an elephant? A piece at a time." I remember that so vividly, and only now do I understand that "a piece at a time" was just as hard for them to say as it was for me to understand.* TRISH

## Symptom Relief

Although the cause of chronic fatigue syndrome (CFS) has not been discovered, we do know that the illness affects many of the body's systems as shown by the vast array of symptoms that people with CFS (PWCFS) experience. When studying the genes of PWCFS, researchers led by Dr. Jonathan Kerr of St. George's University in London found that CFS could be grouped into seven different types (subtypes) that correlate to the illness' symptoms and how severe they are. More research into CFS subtypes must be done to validate these findings, which may then lead to better diagnosis and treatment, including medications that address symptoms more likely to be found within particular subgroups under which someone's illness falls.

### ARE THERE SUBTYPES OF CFS?

When Dr. Kerr and his team of researchers identified seven subtypes of CFS in the genes of PWCFS, they found that all of the subtypes included fatigue. Although more research is needed to validate these findings, the following are the seven subtypes that correlate to the symptoms each demonstrated and how severe they are:

I: Cognitive, musculoskeletal, and sleep-related symptoms, including anxiety and depression (more severe subtype)

II: Musculoskeletal and symptoms related to pain, and anxiety and/or depression (more severe subtype)

III: Mild symptoms

IV: Mainly cognitive symptoms

V: Mainly musculoskeletal and gastrointestinal symptoms

VI: Mainly postexertional malaise (extreme crash after exercise or exertion)

VII: Pain, infections, as well as musculoskeletal, sleep-related, neurologic, gastrointestinal, and neurocognitive symptoms, including anxiety/depression (more severe subtype)

## Matching Medication With Symptoms

At the present time, there are no medications specifically prescribed to cure CFS; rather, medications for CFS are aimed at alleviating the symptoms. PWCFS have a daunting responsibility to learn to analyze the particular symptom they are experiencing in order to know which medication may help alleviate it at the time they are experiencing it. For example, pain is usually not the same on a daily or even hourly basis. It may vary from mild soreness to bone-crushing acuteness. After discriminating the type of pain, the PWCFS can make an appropriate choice of taking a nonsteroidal anti-inflammatory drug (NSAID) like ibuprofen to alleviate the soreness rather than a strong narcotic like codeine (with a risk of greater side effects). Knowing your symptoms is a difficult task (especially when you are not feeling well), and takes time and experience.

Some medications address more than one symptom; for example, analgesics and/or NSAIDs as well as muscle relaxants can be used for pain and often benefit sleep as well. Although it may be more convenient and cost effective to take only one "pill" for two symptoms, this may make the choice regarding which medication to take for which symptom more challenging. PWCFS have to weigh the symptoms with the benefits and possible side effects before taking medications.

# Off-Label Medications

If your health care provider prescribes a medication classified as an antiseizure drug, this may seem confusing if you do not have a seizure disorder. This is an example of an "off-label" medication. Prescribing "off label" is a common medical practice. Your health care provider prescribes the medication for a medical use other than the one that received approval by the Food and Drug Administration (FDA). In other words, these medications have FDA approval for a different use; for example, antiseizure drugs used to control seizures are prescribed to control a person's mood. When health care providers prescribe these to PWCFS, they are doing so "off label" for use as a mood stabilizer.

### MEDICATIONS THAT TARGET CFS SYMPTOMS

The following are some of the types of medications, with examples, that a health care provider may prescribe for CFS symptom relief:

- **Analgesics**
  - ○ **Non-narcotics** (sold over the counter) such as acetaminophen (Tylenol)

- ○ **Narcotics** such as codeine with acetaminophen hydro-codone (Lorcet or Vicodin) for severe pain when needed (with health care provider management)
- **Antiallergy agents** such as astemizole (Hismanal) or lorata-dine (Claritin)
- **Antianxiety agents** for anxiety, such as buspirone (BuSpar), clonazepam (Klonopin), or alprazolam (Xanax), or lorazepam (Ativan)
- **Antidepressants** for depression (but can also help with sleep, low energy levels, and pain)
  - ○ **Tricyclic antidepressants** such as amitriptyline (Elavil, Sinequan), desipramine (Norpramin), nortriptyline (Pamelor), or clomipramine (Anafranil)
  - ○ **Selective serotonin reuptake inhibitors** such as bupro-pion (Wellbutrin), nefazodone (Serzone), or mirtazapine (Remeron)
  - ○ **Serotonin and norepinephrine reuptake inhibitors** such as Cymbalta duloxetine (Cymbalta)
- **Antihypertensives** or β-blockers for high blood pressure, such as atenolol (Tenormin)
- **Antihypotensives** for orthostatic intolerance (dizziness, fainting) such as fludrocortisone (Florinef)
- **Muscle relaxants** for pain and sleep, such cyclobenzaprine (Flexeril) or the antidepressants amitriptyline (Endep)
- **Antiseizure agents** for pain, sleep, and mood stabilization, such as Neurontin (gabapentin), valproic acid (Depakote), car-bamazepine (Tegretol), or topiramate (Topamax)
- **Nonsteroidal anti-inflammatory drugs** such as over-the-coun-ter ibuprofen (Advil, Motrin) or newer prescription NSAIDs such as diclofenac (Voltaren) or the long-acting Voltaren XL, or sulindac (Clinoril) for pain
- **Psychostimulants** for fatigue and cognitive problems such as difficulty concentrating or memory problems, such as amphetamine and dextroamphetamine (Adderall),

## What Nurses Know ...

Ampligen, the first experimental drug tested for treatment of CFS, has a long (thirty-year) history of setbacks regarding FDA approval. Although it is not yet available, PWCFS have participated—and some are currently participating—in clinical trials to test the drug's efficacy. Its action on CFS is uncertain, but researchers believe that it works on the immune system, activating the body's natural antiviral pathways and regulating RNase-L, a substance in the body's cells that attacks viruses. Some physician-researchers have found that the drug has been beneficial for some, but not all patients.

ormethylphenidate (Ritalin), modafinil (Provigil), or armodafanil (Nuvigil)

- **Sleep medications to** initiate or sustain sleep. Some that initiate sleep include zolpidem (Ambien), zaleplon (Sonata), or eszopiclone (Lunesta). Drugs prescribed to extend sleep include Desyrel (Trazodone), mirtazapine (Remeron), gabapentin (Neurontin), pregabalin (Lyrica). Over-the-counter medications including melatonin, the antihistamine (Benadryl), acetaminophen with diphenhydramine HCl, the same ingredient as Benadryl (Tylenol PM) or ibuprofen with diphenhydramine HCl, the same ingredient as Benadryl (Advil PM), or doxylamine (used in Nyquil), valerian root, passion flower, or chamomile

## Balancing Treatment With Side Effects

*My earliest memory of taking medicine for CFS dates back to age eight when I was first diagnosed with CFS. My health care provider prescribed a muscle relaxant for pain, which I still take when I need it. The trick is to know when to take it or a less strong over-the-counter medicine. Two years ago (age 16), when I took this muscle relaxant to relieve back pain and then hopefully go shopping with my mom, I became so tired I dozed off in the car. By the time we arrived at the mall, I had fallen asleep, so she drove us home. I now try to take into account the possible side effects before I take any medicine, especially those to relieve pain. If I need a muscle relaxant for pain, I now stay home and rest.*   MARISSA

Medications can help relieve pain, headache, insomnia, and daytime sleepiness, but they come at the price of side effects. For example, one drug may decrease anxiety but increase appetite and weight gain. Another may decrease pain but increase your daytime drowsiness. You have to balance the benefits with the possible ill effects, and this should be done in consultation with your health care provider. Be aware of what the pros and cons of each medication are before you decide to take it. Also, remember that a drug that one person may take successfully may have an ill effect on someone else.

If you find yourself becoming more tired than usual or in more pain than usual, think of the medications you take and talk with your health care provider to help you find out whether one of these may be the cause. Another possibility may be that one of your medications has lost its effectiveness for you, so that a particular symptom is no longer being addressed. You may have built up a tolerance to a medication that resulted from using it regularly, and therefore you now need an increased amount to produce the same effect.

Know that medications, for example, benzodiazepines, may increase your activity level one day, but can make you sleepy a few days later, so the best way to take them is "as needed" rather than on a daily basis. Discuss how to distinguish between an "as needed" and daily dose with your health care provider. The aim is to take as few medications as possible while continuing to function as best as possible.

PWCFS are sensitive to medications. To minimize side effects, in conjunction with your health care provider, start a medication with small amounts and increase them gradually. Monitor any medication side effects such as weight gain, daytime sleepiness, cognitive dysfunction, or sleep disturbances and discuss them with your health care provider.

> *Much of what PWCFS say about their medications is based on experience. We are creating our own research. For example, my original dose of an antidepressant prescribed by my health care provider for pain and to help me get to sleep was the low dose of 25 mg that most adults take. The hangover feeling I had the next morning alerted me to the fact that something was wrong. Rather than not take the medication, I checked with the health care provider and took the suggested 10 mg dose, which manages my pain and sleep with no ill effects. This was real-life proof that PWCFS need to start with a dose of medication lower than those without CFS.* PAT

## What Nurses Know ...

*Medications are expensive. Many pharmaceutical companies provide medications for free, if you qualify. Ask your health care providers if they have application forms for patient assistance programs that are sponsored by the drug company that makes your medication. They may be able to give you free samples during the application process. If you are too ill to do the paperwork, contact a volunteer agency to help.*

*After years of experimentation, I gained an understanding of what medications worked and what didn't work for me. Wake-promoting medication to combat the fog, sleep promoting agents to get restorative sleep, serotonin and norepinephrine reuptake inhibitor (SNRI) antidepressants to dull the chronic physical pain and keep me out of a state of emotional despair... that's my baseline cocktail, interspersed with "off-label" medications for severe breakthrough pain, migraines, allergies, and infections. The experimentation process has a real impact on one's emotional well-being. The hardest part of being a "guinea pig" is thinking that you've finally found a medication that works only to have it taken away.* TRISH

*I found that safe methods of managing CFS meant treating each symptom, mutually exclusively of each other while managing medications collectively. The migraine prevention medication, which is supposed to be taken at night because it causes drowsiness, had to be taken first thing in the morning with the wake-promoting medication so that when the nighttime pain hit, I wasn't overdosing myself with a cocktail of medications that could depress my central nervous system. It was a series of trial and error, but eventually I developed a medication regimen to proactively prevent flare ups while also leaving room for medication*

## What Nurses Know...

*There is no "magic pill" to cure CFS. PWCFS need to focus on proactive strategies that include a combination of symptom management, coping strategies, activity management/ pacing, and exercise therapy.*

*as needed for breakthrough symptoms...until the winter turned to spring and allergy season set in...and I had to start all over again.* TRISH

With CFS, every individual's path is going to be different. Although it may be frustrating, you may have to try different medications in various combinations and also try supplementing these with alternative therapies, which will be discussed in Chapter 8.

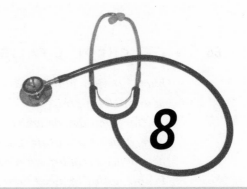

*8*

# Alternative Approaches

*I never fully recovered from Lyme disease. Five years later, I was diagnosed with CFS and fibromyalgia. I couldn't work, but I saw other people with chronic illnesses, like rheumatoid arthritis, working. I began to investigate what I could do to help my body heal. It made sense to me that I needed to address how to get better sleep, nutrition, and mobility. I read about integrative therapies and realized that, just as Chinese medicine says, it's important to try to achieve a sense of balance in life to be healthy and help the body heal. This calls for decisions. For example, to get to sleep at night should I take prescription medications that may cause side effects or learn how to meditate and relax with no downside?*

*I've tried a variety of integrative therapies to increase energy and counter symptoms: Tai Chi, Qigong, acupuncture, acupressure, Rolfing, homeopathy, meditation, massage, and nutritional therapies, to name a few. The decision here is to find out what gives you the "most bang for the buck." Do hot baths and massage, for example, work for your muscle pain?*

*Once you decide which therapies to integrate into your care, develop a routine. I look at this as maintenance. Most people need regular maintenance to function better, longer. People with CFS need more maintenance than the average person.*

*Yes, I still relapse, but I function and am getting on with my life. From time to time, I have to psyche myself up to stay on course.* MARY ELLEN

## Alternative, Complementary, and Integrative Therapies

When our daughter Trish was twelve, she experienced chronic fatigue syndrome (CFS)-related back pain, which was somewhat relieved by acupuncture. When her back pain was acute, the neurologist would allow me to bring her in immediately for trigger point injections with the local anesthetic lidocaine, which would provide her relief for a few hours. Trigger points are knots or bumps of muscle that form when muscles fail to relax. Some might consider these treatments as complementary to her typical medical treatment of CFS symptoms or even alternatives to medical treatment. However, because these treatments had research evidence showing that they were safe and could be effective for CFS symptoms, we integrated them into Trish's plan of care. Again, this integrative medicine is not intended to replace a traditional medical plan of care, rather to complement it.

Before deciding to try a therapy and/or include one in your care, it is important to research it, make sure it has been scientifically tested for safety, discuss it with your health care provider, and then start slowly, paying close attention to how your body responds. Some remedies are harmless, but some may cause side effects. Be careful with misleading advertisements about vitamins, supplements, and what are called "cure all" treatments. If the product "cures all," why are people still ill? At the same time, many "alternative" treatments are being explored and researched by mainstream Western medicine now and are clearly more accepted than they were in the past.

Be clear on what your goal is for the therapy because some may be better than others for your target goal. For example, if your goal is to reduce stress and increase relaxation, body work such as massage therapy might be helpful for you. Massage therapy relaxes the entire body, loosens and relieves tight muscles, diminishes pain, and reduces mental stress. Some therapies that may be helpful to alleviate CFS symptoms are discussed in this chapter.

## Massage

Depending on your symptom, you can choose from various types of massage:

- Swedish massage involves manipulating muscles for relaxation; therapeutic massage such as myofascial release to get muscles and connective tissue to relax and function properly
- Rolfing relies on deep pressure to relax muscles' connective tissues that have become stiff and painful, or neuromuscular massage where pressure is applied to specific muscles to increase blood flow or release tension or pain
- Trigger point therapy involves concentrated finger pressure applied to "trigger points" to relieve muscular pain. The trigger points, according to Chinese medicine, are points along invisible meridians that mark the path of energy through the body.

## Myofascial Release Therapy

Myofascial release therapy is often considered a type of massage. It consists of very gentle manipulation of the fascia (connective tissue located between the skin and underlying structure of muscle and bone). Fascia can become tight and restricted in response to injury, inflammation, stress, or even poor posture. Over time, the tightness in one area can spread throughout the whole body, which can be quite painful. The goal of myofascial release is to release the restricted fascia, which in turn eases the pain, increases the patient's range of motion, and brings the body into balance.

## Yoga

According to the Centers for Disease Control and Prevention, therapies like yoga can be beneficial in reducing anxiety and promoting a sense of well-being. The gentle stretching exercises of yoga, dating back to ancient India, can improve muscle tone, posture, mental clarity, stress control, and relaxation. It involves specific exercises, meditation, and breathing techniques.

*What Nurses Know...*

*When considering a nontraditional therapy, be skeptical of therapies that*

- *proclaim to be a miracle cure*
- *use only testimonials to prove they work*
- *claim they are a secret formula*
- *are advertised in magazines or on TV rather than discussed in medical journals as safe and effective*

Although there are different types of yoga, gentle yoga stretching found in Hatha yoga is encouraged rather than strenuous types of yoga that involve aerobic activity.

## Tai Chi

Tai Chi, also called moving meditation, is a sequence of posture-enhancing, center-of-gravity, slow deliberate movements supported with deep breathing and meditation, aimed to increase energy and flexibility. Tai Chi dates back to thirteenth century China. Although Tai Chi is considered gentle, some people with CFS (PWCFS) may find it too strenuous. Any type of exercise must be individualized. Check with your health care provider before attempting them. Work into them gradually and notice the effect it may be having on your body. To try to avoid postexertional malaise, rest in between Tai Chi movements.

## Biofeedback

Biofeedback uses electrical sensors that are attached to the body to measure physical functions such as pulse and blood pressure. You use the information you receive (feedback) about your body (bio) to make subtle changes such as relaxing certain muscles to achieve the results you want, such as reducing pain or relieving muscle tension and stress. For example, by practicing relaxation techniques and watching how the body reacts via the electronic monitor, you can learn to control body responses. Biofeedback makes users aware that they have the power to gain control of their body processes to increase relaxation and relieve pain and make lasting changes in their bodies and minds.

*I include complementary therapies like Tai Chi Chih, mild yoga, and acupuncture to help manage stiffness and pain. Tai Chi Chih is similar to Tai Chi, but not based on martial arts. It's slow, effortless movement that doesn't cause stress to the body. I feel that it strengthens my muscles and improves my balance. It's like a moving meditation.* NANCY

## Acupuncture

Acupuncture, a Chinese therapy dating back more than 2,000 years, incorporates very thin needles inserted into invisible meridian points on certain areas of the body. Acupuncturists treat people based on an individualized assessment of the excesses and deficiencies of energy (Qi) located on the various meridians. The needles stimulate the points that balance the person's energy and help the body heal. Acupuncture is used to relieve pain and nausea. Some evidence also suggests that acupuncture may help boost the immune system, and may help PWCFS get a more restful night's sleep.

## Homeopathy

Homeopathy makes use of natural pharmaceuticals, derived from plants, minerals, and animals, to create similar symptoms a person is experiencing so that the body can build its own defenses and heal itself. Practitioners certified by the American Board of Homeotherapeutics and National Standards provide

## What Nurses Know . . .

*With homeopathy, the smallest amount needed to stimulate the immune system is given, and there is no one dose; it is all individually determined.*

these products as part of a personal care plan to patients. In the United States, twelve states recognize licensed homeopathic practitioners and only three states license physicians to practice homeopathy. Advocates of homeopathy refer to immunizations in traditional medicine and how they encourage the body to develop antibodies to protect against disease to support homeopathy.

## Mindfulness-Based Stress Reduction

Mindfulness-based stress reduction (MBSR) uses mindfulness meditation to improve well-being and alleviate suffering. This technique of meditation fosters awareness of the present moment. The first formal MBSR program was developed by Jon Kabat-Zinn in the 1990s as an eight-week program that includes formal mindfulness meditation, education on mental and physical stress response, and group support. Research has shown MBSR to be beneficial for people with chronic illnesses, including fibromyalgia and CFS.

## Therapeutic Touch

Therapeutic touch (TT) was developed in the 1970s by Dora Kunz, a theosophy promoter, and Dolores Krieger, PhD, RN, a nursing educator at New York University. TT is an energy medicine intervention based on both Eastern and Western physical science. Practitioners intentionally direct energy exchange by placing their hands near the patient to detect their energy field and facilitate healing. The receiver is not usually touched and may not even be in the same room; rather, the practitioner's intention of directing healing energy may enable the person to heal. TT practitioners believe that they are conduits who can influence healing energy or the vital life energy that surrounds and interpenetrates the physical body. Although some studies show that TT is effective, for example, for relieving pain and improving quality of life in people with fibromyalgia and for decreasing pain and stiffness in arthritic knees, research results are mixed. More studies need to be done to show effectiveness for CFS symptom relief.

# Chiropractic

Chiropractic care is a form of health care that focuses on the relationship between the body's structure, primarily of the spine, and its function. Chiropractors use a type of hands-on therapy called manipulation. They suggest that spinal manipulation may boost energy and decrease pain in some PWCFS. They believe that spinal manipulation may have a stimulating effect on the nervous system. Chiropractic care works on the theory that vitality and good health are due to an unobstructed flow of nerve impulses from the brain through the spinal nerves and throughout the rest of the body. When misalignments or "subluxations" occur, such as joint dysfunctions, joint adhesions, or joint fixations, there is an interference with the normal transmission of nerve impulses. If this continues over a long period of time, there is impaired capability, often accompanied by pain. A chiropractor uses "adjustments"–quick, forceful movements–to change the range of joint movement back to normal.

# Osteopathy

Osteopathy is different from chiropractic manipulation, because it focuses on the entire musculoskeletal system rather than just the spine. Osteopathic treatment consists of very gentle and subtle manipulations of the body and sometimes includes cranial work with the bones and membrane attachments in the head.

## Physical Therapy

Long thought of as a rehabilitation science, physical therapy is now used to treat a wide range of conditions, from car accidents to injuries caused by strenuous exercise to stiffness and mobility problems. CFS fits into the category of conditions that might respond to physical therapy; however, consult your health care provider before making an appointment. A physical therapist may prescribe the use of specific functional training and therapeutic exercise, as well as the application of heat, cold, ultrasound, and/or electrical stimulation. The physical therapist must be very knowledgeable about the illness. Care is to be taken to avoid overactivity and the resulting postexertional malaise.

> *My non-traditional, alternative therapy is swimming. Twenty-five years ago I started taking an Aquacise class to keep my arthritic joints moving. When I developed CFS, I just kept swimming. I could no longer walk to the cafeteria with my friends after class, but I was fine in the water. In the water, I'm the me I was before I was ill. After each hour-long swim, I feel refreshed—not fatigued. It is not just the physical effort; it is also the tranquility and peace that is so relaxing and energizing. When I get out of the pool, it's an effort to walk, but the peace remains.* PAT

## A Word About Herbs and Supplements

Frustration with CFS symptoms and the inability for relief from traditional medications may encourage PWCFS to try herbs and supplements. PWCFS may think that "natural" remedies will offer a gentler relief without side effects. Natural, however, doesn't necessarily mean safe.

Herbs are chemicals too and can cause ill effects. Herbal remedies do not often undergo the same type of scientific testing as conventional drugs. There can be question as to the effectiveness of the herb as well as the resulting side effects when taken with conventional medication.

Although research has shown the effectiveness of the over-the-counter herbal remedy—St. John's wort for depression—when taken with prescribed antidepressant medications like Prozac or Paxil, side effects like tremor, anxiety, mental status change, restlessness, and headache can occur. At this time, we do not have any solid evidence that supplements do help alleviate symptoms of CFS.

Supplements may produce modest improvement in some symptoms for some people. Before he recommends a supplement to his CFS patients, Dr. Charles Lapp, the director of the Hunter-Hopkins Center in Charlotte, NC, says that the supplement must be safe, have a scientific basis for its use, and must produce a positive effect in at least fifty percent of people who use it. He has found six useful supplements for his patients with CFS:

- A multivitamin that includes B complex, folate, vitamin D, calcium and magnesium
- B12, injectable form
- Vitamin D3 with the dosage of 2,000 units per day
- Calcium 1,000 mg to 1,500 mg daily and magnesium 500 to 750 mg daily (inappropriate for those with kidney disease and may cause diarrhea), which can be taken together in a calcium-magnesium tablet
- D-ribose with the dosage of 5,000 mg three times daily for two weeks, followed by 5,000 mg twice daily; check results, which are obvious within three weeks

If you decide to take herbs or supplements, start only one new one at a time. Then wait a week or two before introducing another one. That will give you a chance to see what effect each

## What Nurses Know...

*Some herbs and complementary and alternative therapies may cause interactions with traditional medications. Health care providers should be made aware when PWCFS use them. If undergoing surgery, it is especially important for the anesthesiologist to know of any therapies. The American Society of Anesthesiologists recommends that all herbal medications be discontinued two to three weeks beforehand to avoid ill effects.*

supplement has on your body. If you do not notice a difference in symptoms, do not continue taking the supplement.

Also, on a note about anesthesia, PWCFS are more sensitive, warranting lower doses. When it comes to surgery, they must be wary of anesthesia. The New Jersey Chronic Fatigue Syndrome Association, Inc., provides cards called ANESTHESIA WARNING for PWCFS about to have surgery. The cards describe what anesthesiologists should do for them because of their heightened sensitivity to anesthesia.

For more information go to www.njcfsa.org.

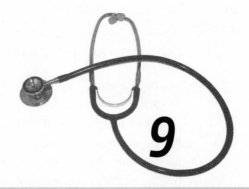

**9**

# The Importance of Advocacy

*It's so upsetting not to be able to function day after day after day. I don't want to feel sorry for myself. My attitude is the one thing I have control over and can work on, and it makes a big difference in my life. It's a daily battle. I won't say I always win, but I do most of the time. I've found that if I get the right group of friends, talk to people, go out for lunch with them once a week, it's not as stressful.*   MARYANNE

Advocacy begins within. As MaryAnne points out, people with chronic fatigue syndrome (PWCFS) do not have control over how they will feel physically, but they can choose a positive attitude and be advocates for themselves or, especially in down times, allow people to advocate for them. If you are a person with chronic fatigue syndrome (CFS), rather than looking at CFS as controlling you, realize that you control your own circumstances. This leads to empowerment and the ability to advocate for yourself.

Many people find it difficult to ask others to do something for them. When people have a chronic illness such as CFS, it makes sense to advocate for oneself by speaking up and asking for assistance. For example, the person with CFS who knows that she will catch a cold when she sits under a draft at work can either put up with the draft or advocate for herself and ask for a desk change or have the air vent closed.

Advocacy means collaborating with others to get your needs met to manage your illness and rebuild your lives. PWCFS require substantial support as evidenced by the stories PWCFS tell and have published. Researchers who looked at studies containing stories of 2,500 patients with CFS found that the major support needs that PWCFS have talked or written about include the need to

- make sense of symptoms and gain diagnosis
- have respect and empathy from service providers
- have positive attitudes and support from family and friends
- obtain information on CFS
- adjust views and priorities
- develop strategies to manage impairments and activity limitations
- develop strategies to maintain or regain social participation

Family, caregivers, friends, health care providers, support groups, CFS organizations, and professional advocates such as attorneys form a wide umbrella under which PWCFS can stand for protection and support.

The need to make sense of symptoms and gain a diagnosis are crucial early in the onset of the illness. Not having a diagnosis may lead to a lack of self-esteem or to feelings of uncertainty. PWCFS may become frightened and wonder why their body seems to be failing them. The lack of a diagnosis can be challenging to friends and family who cannot understand why their loved one looks so well but seems to be ill frequently or to be withdrawing from activities. Family and friends who are first on the scene can become the initial advocates who support PWCFS, encourage them to seek medical attention, and keep up with a social life as much as possible.

Supportive advocates can encourage them to avoid those who do not offer support and to continue to seek health care providers who are supportive. If well-meaning family members or uninformed health care providers encourage patients to do more than they are able, patient advocates may encourage them to pace themselves and seek out other medical opinions.

Advocates can help PWCFS navigate through the health care system and find a knowledgeable, caring health care provider. They may offer their services to drive people to medical appointments. When necessary, they may help PWCFS report their most pressing problems, ask appropriate questions, and take notes about the doctor's recommendations and comments. Advocates can also help people living with CFS when they have difficulty performing everyday duties like doing the laundry or grocery shopping, and make suggestions on how to make life easier, for example, keeping important items like car keys in the same place all the time.

PWCFS and their advocates can seek out the information they need about the illness and how to manage everyday life from knowledgeable health care providers, nurses, occupational or physical therapists, books, newsletters, conferences about CFS, and educational organizations. PWCFS can empower themselves through knowledge gained on reputable Web sites that contribute to their overall treatment and wellness. The Resource section of this book provides lists of reputable Web sites, organizations, and newsletters.

*Of course, I'd do anything for my children. Inherently, parents are their children's advocates, but when it comes to having a child with CFS, advocacy takes on a unique role. It means being the parent who protects, champions, supports, and encourages in the context of a chronic illness. It means learning all you can about CFS, beating down the doors of health care providers to obtain the attention the child needs, fighting with your energy because your child has none. All this for love and the child's better quality of life.* LORRAINE

Advocates offer physical and emotional support by

- keeping an open line of communication by being nonjudgmental toward both patients and the professionals with whom they must collaborate
- validating PWCFS, by confirming the belief that they have a serious illness, even if a health care provider shows doubt; then offering to help find a supportive health care provider.
- asking PWCFS what they need and how they can help
- listening rather than providing suggestions on how to "fix" things
- offering support and understanding when PWCFS cancel plans due to illness or fatigue
- offering positive responses such as, "I'm sorry you're feeling so bad" or "You're handling things so well," or "I know this is difficult for you"
- avoiding comments such as, "You can beat this thing, if you try hard;" avoiding negative comparisons such as, "You walked for a longer time yesterday" or "You used to have such energy"

*In 1997, I experienced the typical CFS symptoms like fatigue and sore throat, but my main problem was dizziness. It took almost two years until an eye ear nose and throat (EENT) specialist diagnosed me with chronic EBV, which he later called CFS. I had to make changes and work from home. Having a chronic illness like CFS means making lifestyle modifications. If you're a Type A personality like I was, you learn to ratchet it down a notch.*

*Advocacy also helps. First you have to advocate for your health. You need a health care provider who understands you; if not, find another who's sympathetic. You don't need "friends" or relatives who belittle you. Negative thinking is stressful, so limit your time with negative people. Next, you can help others advocate for themselves. I became involved with a CFS Support Group and the NJCFSA, which has been a very positive, supporting experience.*

*Life is not the same as it used to be. I used to love to ski and roller blade. I've learned to reengineer my life into a life that's rewarding, not disabling.* NANCY

The nature of CFS can make it difficult for people to vigorously engage in advocacy efforts for themselves. Your local or national CFS advocacy groups are crucial in these cases, as professional organizations have the energy and skill to make a difference as far as the politics of this disease go.

*I gave a presentation at a New Jersey Chronic Fatigue Syndrome Association (NJCFSA) Conference once about growing up with CFS, all the trials and tribulations. It was a comic strip of my life called, "Sometimes All You Can Do is Laugh." And that's the truth…at the end of the day, you have to find the strength to laugh at the insanity so that it doesn't defeat you. I dedicated the comic strip to my mom because she gave me life twice: first when I was born, then again when she got it back for me through her unwavering support in advocating for me when I couldn't do it for myself.* TRISHA

## Advocacy for Children

Children cannot adequately express how they feel, so parents must think of all possibilities and ask them questions to draw out and piece together the health puzzle. When they complain that they are tired, their bones hurt, and they just do not feel well, you might think they are involved in too many activities, are staying up too late, are having a growth spurt, or any number of things. When your twelve-year-old child does not want to get up and go to school, what do you do? She says she is so tired, she cannot move. She does not seem to have a fever. The day before, she seemed fine. You give her a day to "feel better," but the same thing happens again. She cannot get out of bed. Do you think there must be something wrong at school? Force her to get up and go to school? Take her to the doctor?

When this scenario played out with my twelve-year-old daughter Trisha, I brought her to the pediatrician on the second day. I did not think of CFS, but I became her parent/patient advocate who walked her through the health care system until we finally got a diagnosis about a year later.

It is difficult being an advocate for children because they may feel guilty that they are so tired all the time and, therefore, may not complain. Unable to remember what it feels like to have energy, they may begin to think it is normal to always feel tired. Some children's complaints are inconsistent. Sometimes they complain of sore throat, pain, and dizziness that is disabling. Next time, they complain of dizziness and may not have all the "right" symptoms at the right time for a medical diagnosis.

Children who have these kinds of problems are often overlooked, thought to be depressed, considered school-avoidant or irresponsible, lazy, lacking ambition or energy, or are self-centered. As advocates, parents must take their children seriously, listen to what they have to say, and seek medical attention. Not believing children creates a web of doubt within them, making them doubt what they feel, think, and know. Believing in your child is the first step toward obtaining a correct diagnosis, treatment, and better quality of life.

## What Nurses Know...

*CFS in children has been trivialized, believed to be short-lived in children, and sometimes thought to be a manifestation of psychiatric problems. Although it is possible that CFS can be mild and resolve completely in some children, in many there is a wide spectrum of illness severity that includes functional limitation and severe pain. There is an urgent need for increased attention to CFS (as a serious, sometimes life-threatening illness) among children, one that cannot be denied or explained away by psychiatric theory.*

## Advocacy in School

CFS causes major disruption in the education of children. Parents can be advocates for their children by learning about the educational needs of their children and how to get these needs fulfilled. They can obtain information from sources such as the National Information Center for Children and Youth with Disabilities about disabilities, children's rights, and the individualized education plans (IEPs) for school.

Under the Individuals with Disabilities Education Act (IDEA) and/or accommodations under Section 504 of the Rehabilitation Act of 1973, children who are disabled by CFS are entitled to special educational services. The IDEA mandates a free and appropriate public education for all children with disabilities. If the children are at a preillness level and ineligible for services under IDEA, they may be entitled to educational accommodations under Section 504 of the Rehabilitation Act of 1973, which assures them equal opportunities through accommodations written into an IEP aimed to help children participate and benefit from the educational program.

## What Nurses Know...

School nurses are advocates for all students, especially those who are challenged with CFS. To help children with CFS have as normal a life as possible both in and out of school time, school nurses recommend that

- care may be directed by out-of-area doctors, due to the limited number of CFS specialists
- physical education and school activities (if medically advised and self-limiting) should be considered as a child's vital part of social development
- teachers be alerted that postactivity days (physical education, etc.) may require students to stay home and rest the next day or more
- students with CFS alternate in-school days with home tutoring days as needed and prescribed by their health care provider
- students with CFS may need to arrive late to school to allow for a natural wake-up cycle (as recommended by their health care provider)
- students with CFS may qualify for Honors classes, but may still need accommodations
- students with CFS may need in-school rest and snack time, and should be permitted to carry a bottle of water with them
- students with CFS be given a second set of books for home use.

PAT LAROSA, RN, MSN, School Nurse

If the child with CFS meets IDEA's disability classification of "other health impaired" defined by "...limited strength, vitality or alertness, due to chronic or acute health problems, which adversely affects a child's educational performance," the parents and Child Study Team (guidance counselor, principal, and teachers) meet to develop the IEP, which is reviewed and updated annually or as needed. The success of the IEP depends on teamwork; failure results with one unwilling person.

*In high school, I had a first-year teacher for AP English. I'd been out for three days, and did not have my literature book at home. When I returned to school, I sat down in English class and was presented with a test on the material covered while I was out sick. I pleaded with the teacher, saying that I was out sick and didn't have the book at home, there was no way I could have prepared for the exam. He said, "Trisha this is an honors English class. You are expected*

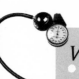

## What Nurses Know...

*Examples of accommodations for children with an IEP, developed in conjunction with the school Child Study Team, teachers, and parents may include*

- *school tutors at home*
- *longer time for test taking*
- *untimed tests for Scholastic Achievement Tests for college admission*
- *longer due dates for assignments*
- *ability to tape-record lessons*
- *student-buddy to help with note-taking*
- *seating in front of the class*
- *special bus pick-up*
- *extra set of books to remain at home*
- *passes to use the school elevator and to visit the nurse's office as needed*

*to keep up." As I submitted my blank exam, I reminded him that I had an IEP. He said that he couldn't let things slide because it set an unfair precedent to the other students. "Come on, Trisha, I'm teaching an honors class. I have to retain the reputation of a 'hard-ass'." Trying to keep back my tears, I said, "When you discriminate against sick kids, you gain the reputation of an 'ass-hole'."* TRISHA

*As a patient diagnosed with CFS/ME and fibromyalgia (FM), I quickly came to the realization that advocacy would play an important role in my life. Without someone willing to stand up for an adequate and better quality of life for those with disabilities meant that I would merely be a survivor, not having the ability to thrive and succeed. I decided that someone had to be me.* MARLY SILVERMAN, FOUNDER OF P.A.N.D.O.R.A.

## Reaching Out

Advocacy also means reaching out, forming or joining groups, and becoming active to achieve what is needed for PWCFS. For example, Marly Silverman, diagnosed with CFS, founded P.A.N.D.O.R.A. (the Patient Alliance for Neuroendocrineimmune Disorders Organizations, Inc.) to assist patients with neuroendocrineimmune disorders and their families in leading productive and fulfilling lives. The organization aims to create and raise awareness, advocate for quality of life issues, provide support and educational resources, establish partnerships in the worldwide community, support scientific research, encourage creation of empowerment groups, and organize educational conferences. P.A.N.D.O.R.A., also known as PANDORA, has spearheaded campaigns to increase research funding for CFS and related Neuroendocrineimmune diseases and establish centers for clinical training of primary care physicians for the proper diagnosis and treatment of CFS. One of its campaigns includes a patient-driven and physician-approved project to establish the Neuroendocrineimmune Center in New Jersey and Florida, which will be the first research center dedicated to understanding multisystem, chronic and complex diseases, and treating them effectively.

Local CFS organizations, such as the New Jersey Chronic Fatigue Syndrome Association (NJCFSA) founded by former CFS patient Jon Sterling, offer support groups, conferences, lending libraries with books, articles, video tapes and DVDs, health care provider and attorney referrals, and interaction with other CFS organizations. They are made up of PWCFS, their families, and friends who are advocates ready to support, inform, and help people cope with CFS. The NJCFSA advocates at the state level and produced and distributed the *A Consensus Manual for the Primary Care and Management of Chronic Fatigue Syndrome* to NJ physicians. The manual has been translated into Spanish and Japanese.

Advocacy by the Vermont CFIDS Association resulted in a bill passed to educate primary care physicians and other health care providers in that state about CFS. The bill allowed for the printing and distribution of the *A Consensus Manual for the Primary Care and Management of Chronic Fatigue Syndrome* to Vermont health care providers, in conjunction with the Vermont Department of Health.

There are national advocacy organizations such as the CFIDS Association of America and the IACFS/ME (International Association for Chronic Fatigue Syndrome/ ME). The CFIDS Association of America funds research, provides information, and employs a lobbying organization, the Sheridan Group, to look out for ME/CFS patients' interests on Capitol Hill.

In 1998, after CFIDS Association of America President Kim McCleary asked a Centers for Disease Control and Prevention (CDC) official how the $22.7 million Congress authorized for

ME/CFS research was being spent, it was discovered that nearly $13 million of the funding was diverted to research in other areas. The CDC was directed to replace the money. The CFIDS Association of America annual Lobby Day and Grassroots advocacy center provide patients the opportunity to participate in federal advocacy.

The International Association of CFS/ME (IACFS/ME) has been active under the leadership of Dr. Nancy Klimas and lobbies for PWCFS, but has no paid staff members. The group provides biannual international conferences, a free newsletter, and sponsored the recent pediatric definition of CFS. The IACFS/ME is raising funds to hire its first staff member and is currently creating treatment guidelines for this disease.

## Advocating for Disability Insurance Benefits

*No one ever wants to be on disability. People have told me, "You have it easy; you don't have to work." They have no idea what it means not to work and collect a pay check. I'm blessed because I have social security benefits, but it puts me in a vulnerable situation. Financially, I'm below the poverty line. At age 45, I wonder what will happen long-term when my savings are gone. Will I lose my house? Will I ever be well enough to work again?* STEVE

Under social security law, people are considered disabled when they are unable to do any substantial gainful work activity because of a medical condition that has lasted, or can be expected to last, for at least twelve months, or that is expected to result in death. In the case of those younger than eighteen years, they must have any medically determinable physical or mental impairment that results in marked and severe functional limitations. CFS is a medically determinable impairment that can be the basis for disability; however, according to the

Social Security Administration, all claims must be accompanied by medical signs or laboratory findings. In the case of CFS, people living with CFS who need disability insurance benefits must provide supporting evidence that they qualify.

The Social Security Administration requires the following detailed information from physicians of PWCFS who are applying for disability insurance benefits:

- Medical reports with medical history, clinical and laboratory findings with copies of these results and results of any mental status exams
- Physician records containing detailed historical notes that discuss the course of CFS, including treatment and response
- Physician's opinion statement regarding what work-related activities the PWCFS can still do despite impairment with descriptions of any functional limitations noted

An adjudication team consisting of a physician or psychologist and a specially trained disability examiner working in the disability determination services in the State in which the claimant lives evaluates the PWCFS.

*At 25 years of age, I didn't think I would ever need disability insurance. The "mental battle" of getting disability benefits was difficult for me. I came to terms with it because it's another way of survival—to be able to get medical help and pay the bills.*   STEVE

Because there are no "objective" tests to prove someone has CFS, PWCFS can use other means to show that they are ill, and to the extent that they need disability insurance benefits. In addition to health care providers' reports (as mentioned earlier), PWCFS should keep a journal to describe their symptoms and the progression of their illness including how performing tasks affects them.

The length of time it takes for approval for disability insurance benefits varies. If denied, PWCFS can appeal the decision. CFS organizations and support groups can be guides for this process, and for finding attorneys when needed.

*At a time in your life when all you want to do is sleep and you're so tired you don't want to get out of bed, you must be organized and keep records to successfully apply for disability benefits.* STEVE

## What Nurses Know . . .

*Tips to help PWCFS file for disability insurance benefits*

- *Find a health care provider who is knowledgeable about and believes in CFS and in you.*
- *Keep a journal or diary of your CFS symptoms, including a timeline of the progression of your illness.*
- *Keep all medical records and receipts in a folder or in a separate box.*
- *Use resources: a support group as a guide through the process, an attorney when need be, and your State senator as a liaison between you and the Social Security Administration Office.*
- *Be persistent.*

*These tips are suggested by Steve, a person living with chronic fatigue syndrome.

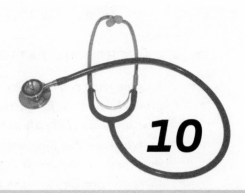

10

# Looking Ahead: Living With Chronic Illness

*In order to explain my life with CFS, I need to describe how it was before. Since childhood I've had rheumatoid arthritis, so I learned long ago that there is life after illness...*if you choose it.

*I had always been a "goer" and a "doer." I had lots of energy, three grown children, a tidy home, and the hopes of becoming a grandmother. When I developed CFS, I was halfway through my graduate work for a Master's in Nursing. It was an online program, so I did my reading and papers lying down on my bed. I would get up to type them into my computer, print them out, and return to bed to edit. The horizontal position helped keep my thoughts clear.*

*I continue to "go" and "do," but at a somewhat modified pace. I work as a substitute school nurse and manage my precious energy by staggering my schedule to have at least one rest day between work days. I spend time with my grandchildren. In fact, I have had 10 grandchildren in the first six years of my life with CFS.*

*When my daughter was on bed rest during her second pregnancy, I alternated days with her mother-in-law to be there to care for her two-year-old. Yes, I often spent the interim days in bed, dreading that I would even have to get up to go to the bathroom. But life is so worth it!*

*I am an optimist by nature and accept what is. I have adapted my life so I can feel fulfilled. Being involved in helping others with CFS adds to that satisfaction. Not every day is easy, but that is part of life.* PAT

The challenge of having chronic fatigue syndrome (CFS) means learning to live day to day with a chronic illness. This challenge is different for each person because CFS affects people differently. The course of the illness varies among individuals. Although some people with CFS (PWCFS) become disabled, others rally and carry on life with an "almost as if I never had CFS" ability.

## Recovery?

Do people recover from CFS? Relating recovery with CFS brings with it more questions than answers. What do you mean by recovery? Do you mean a complete return to how you were before CFS?

Complete recovery remains uncertain. According to the Centers for Disease Control (CDC), the limited research available appears to point toward a five-year improvement rate after the onset of CFS. If the symptoms last for five years, it is unlikely that CFS will improve significantly as time goes on. The studies are limited and because people are individuals, the response to illness varies.

Some patients recover after two to four years, while others remain ill for decades. Recovery and/or remission is in the range of five to ten percent. Researchers have found some factors that provide a better prognosis for patients whose symptoms began abruptly with mild fatigue and those who do not have a psychiatric illness. According to CDC researcher James Jones, MD, patients who were ill for two years or less (in his studies) were more likely to improve. The longer a person was ill before diagnosis, the more complicated the course of the illness appeared to be.

CFS pediatrician and noted CFS researcher David Bell, MD, and colleagues found more encouraging results in a thirteen-year follow-up study of adolescents who were diagnosed with CFS as children. They found that 80% were better or much better, and only twenty percent were the same or worse as time went by.

Based on his research both in his native Australia and in the United States, Andrew Lloyd, Visiting Research Fellow at the Laboratory of Molecular Immunoregulation, National Cancer Institutes, affirms that recovery is a realistic hope. By recovery, Lloyd means that there is no evidence in the blood or body of any disorder, as he found in his research.

Researcher Phil Peterson, MD, of the University of Minnesota Medical School and Hennepin County Medical Center in Minneapolis, also found results to reinforce this optimistic perspective. Peterson says, "Although CFS waxes and wanes (patients) generally head slowly out of the woods with this illness. Recovery is ... clearly the rule in the majority of patients ..." Peterson says that patients do recover gradually.

These controversial findings may be linked to the fact that research is scarce when it comes to describing the recovery process and how, if, and why some people recover. Until recently, more research has gone into the CFS syndrome and its cause, says William Collinge, PhD, of Collinge and Associates, an independent research and consulting organization funded by the National Institutes of Health to develop innovative approaches to benefiting public health. Collinge, who has written about three phases of CFS—onset, acute phase, and recovery phase—explains the recovery phase as a gradual upward ascent toward health along with CFS symptom relapses and remission of varying degrees. During this recovery phase, the relapses generally become less severe, of less duration, and the time between relapses lengthens. However, relapses can still occur after the person with CFS has recovered a satisfactory level of functioning.

Because treatment is symptom based rather than on elimination of a cause, the majority of PWCFS live with some degree of the illness. In their study of sixty-five PWCFS over a three-year time period, researcher Rosane Nisenbaum and colleagues found that unrefreshing sleep continued in at least 79% of people, but tended to be less frequent over time. Of the small group of PWCFS, 20%-33% had CFS at follow-up but more than half experienced partial or total remission.

The CDC's statistics for full remission (not recovery) stand at four percent. PWCFS recover and then relapse, sometimes years later. Because of the relapsing nature of CFS, there is no consensus about what recovery is.

The term "in recovery" might be appropriate for PWCFS who, like Pat, are not how they were before CFS but have the ability to get on with their lives.

Estimates are that 80% of patients do not get better. According to U.S. statistics provided by the CDC, only four percent of patients had full remission (not recovery) at 24 months.

*Because of CFS, I've learned that I can't be perfect. I used to be a high achiever. The strength I once used to be the high achiever, I now use to get by day by day.* STEVE

# Chronic Illness Model and CFS

During a visit to the pediatrician for a school physical, the doctor looked at my daughter Trisha's chart and asked, "chronic fatigue syndrome—you still have that?" Trish and I just looked at each other in amazement. "Didn't she understand the meaning of the word chronic?"

While attending the New Jersey Chronic Fatigue Syndrome Association-sponsored CFS conference, my husband and I learned what chronic illness means in terms of CFS. Guest speaker and CEO of Albany Health Management Associates, Patricia Fennell, MSW, LCSWR, provided us with invaluable insights into living with CFS as a chronic illness. In addition to the fact that CFS usually lasts an indefinite amount of time, this chronic illness is difficult to treat and manage because it affects many of the body systems often at the same time. In our society, cultural issues compound these physical issues because the U.S. culture has an intolerance to illnesses that lasts as compared to acute illnesses where people get better in a certain timeframe.

Ms. Fennell discussed the Fennell Four-Phase Model, which we used to relate each of the four phases of the model (crisis, stabilization, resolution, and integration) to what Trisha was or would be experiencing with CFS or would cycle through back and forth. Here is how we related Trisha's experience with each phase:

1. Crisis: Trisha came down with Epstein-Barr virus and did not fully recover. She was exhausted and could not return to school. She felt depressed, and experienced the ups and downs of multiple CFS symptoms. (Ms. Fennell said that the crisis phase can go on for years.)
2. Stabilization: Trisha did not feel better, but somewhat learned to deal with her symptoms. She saw many specialists and had counseling to help her deal with her family and people not prepared to cope with a chronic illness. She would appear to

get better, but something would cause a relapse and she would sometimes experience a worsening of symptoms.

3. Resolution: With help, Trisha began to cope with the idea of CFS as part of her life. Rather than the things that she lost through the years, the piano or dance recitals of her childhood, she focused on getting through the day and then the next day. Where she once thought of CFS as a life sentence, she told me that she now sees it as a lifestyle that forces her to pace herself and value each day, each moment. (Ms. Fennell said that people can experience a crisis of the soul and have difficulty coping with the idea of CFS being their life. With help, they need to grieve for their former lives and develop reasons for their story.)

4. Integration: Although it has been difficult not to view relapse as a failure, Trisha began to realize that relapse and recovery are part of having CFS. She now views life as a balancing act; she does the harder tasks when she is feeling well and saves the simpler ones for when she is too fatigued to focus on more difficult ones. (Ms. Fennell said that PWCFS can learn that relapse is a dress rehearsal for getting better.)

The most difficult but eye-opening realization that struck me was that Trisha did indeed have a chronic illness, meaning it will always be there in some shape or form. Our little girl would never again be the same as she was before CFS. Somehow I had secretly (unknown even to myself) had the inkling of hope that she would wake up one day and it would be totally gone.

As discouraging as chronicity appeared, Ms. Fennell gave us hope when she said that PWCFS can come to the phase of redefining themselves each day. I believe that this is what Trisha is doing; however, I still struggle with this. Although it has been more than ten years since Trisha's diagnosis, I still find myself forgetting that she, now an adult, has CFS. When I invite her to go shopping at the mall, for example, she quickly reminds me that it is better for her to shop at one small store rather than at a mall—and this, only when she is up to going shopping.

> *I was going to go with my mom [to a CFS conference], but I couldn't get out of bed. Up until that day, my dad acted towards me with frustration. I knew he wasn't angry at me, but angry that I was sick and scared for me. He didn't understand CFS and felt like his role in my life was that of a worried outsider looking in, watching everything spin out of control.*
>
> *Going to that conference was a turning point for our relationship. He got home, came to my room, and tried not to cry at my bedside while he told me that he was so sorry he hadn't been there to support me; he just didn't understand what I was going through. Having heard the speakers at the conference, he understood it as best a person who doesn't have CFS could.*
>
> *I realized that my having CFS means my whole family has CFS. In the same way that I had to assume a new role, that of a chronically ill person with CFS and fibromyalgia, my family members also had to learn new roles.* TRISHA

## Getting on With One's Life

Even without CFS, life is a balancing act where people with the illness must take precautions to maintain their level of well-being and avoid symptom flare-ups as best they can. Flare-ups can mean increased brain fogginess, muscle or joint pain, or flu-like symptoms, which can last for hours, days, or months. It is possible for PWCFS to figure out what may sometimes trigger a flare-up for them and try to avoid it.

For some people, getting more rest is a large part of the equation for flare-up avoidance. To others, this sounds almost offensive because they do not get restorative sleep, so no matter how much rest they get, it will never seem enough. Thomas, who suffered through CFS symptoms as a child, notices that not getting enough sleep is one of the triggers for symptom flares, so he pencils in rest around work and events and tries to adopt a reasonable schedule.

> *I don't remember much of being diagnosed with CFS as a ten-year-old, but I do remember having bouts with fevers that spiked to 103° F and fatigue that sapped my strength. It was the worst feeling. I was too tired to do anything except occasionally watch TV. It's 16 years later and I feel I'm pretty much recovered. I do get flare-ups of fatigue and fever that can last for a few days if I miss sleep, get run down, or catch a cold or virus.* THOMAS

## Helpful Advice From PWCFS

PWCFS have often had to learn the hard way as to what works and what does not work for them to maintain wellness to the best of their ability. The following are some of their suggestions:

- Listen to your body. Do not exert yourself on days when you feel good. Giving into this temptation may lead to a flare-up.
- Even on good days, pace yourself and take rest breaks—when you have a dinner engagement, for example, but find that dinner is your worst time of the day, consider taking a rest break before dinner, which may regenerate you enough to keep and enjoy the date.
- Things beyond your control, like bad weather, can trigger flare-ups. In this case, the old adage "dressing for the weather" can make a difference. Because many PWCFS are sensitive to cold, they should keep a sweater handy and avoid drafty places. Try to nip a cold in the bud lest it trigger CFS symptoms.

- Stress can drain your energy. When feeling stressed, it helps to look at your life and identify the culprit, which is the first step toward eliminating it.
- Try talking to a good friend or counselor, or practice relaxation techniques like yoga or meditation.
- Find support from a group, a phone buddy, an e-mail buddy, or at an online support group.
- Maintain your friendships by phone, especially when you are too tired to go out.

*Attitude is huge. Smiling and laughing are part of enjoying life, the new life you define after you become ill. It isn't all downhill. It may not be what one planned, but it can be an exciting, happy, and fulfilling life.* PAT

CFS can take its toll on the relationships with family and friends. Because PWCFS look well, even the people closest to them may not realize, forget, or deny that there is anything wrong. This can cause stress during a time when PWCFS need support. Forming a network of support, people can help PWCFS feel less isolated and cope better; however, these friends and family need to know the basics of the illness and what the patient needs.

Good communication where participants really listen to each other and ask for clarification to avoid misunderstanding can help bridge the knowledge gap between PWCFS, family, and friends. When it is a good time for discussions, all parties can ask what they can do for each other. For example, PWCFS can make their needs known by saying, "This would make my life easier. Would you be able to do this for me?" To lessen their difficulty of asking for help, family and friends can ask, "What is something I can do to make your life easier?" PWCFS and families can carve out a convenient time for regular dialogue and problem-solving sessions. CFS brings dramatic change to the person as well as to loved ones. Talking about issues can help patients, families, and friends adjust to the "new normal," a different but best quality of life possible.

> *Someone asked me once how to live with a chronic illness. I told them that as depressing as it sounds, the first step is to come to terms with the fact that you're never going to get better. When you search for answers to unanswerable questions...you don't realize it, but you're wasting precious energy allowing your brain and emotions to argue with your body. You can't fight with your body because you'll exhaust yourself, and you'll lose. You have to go through a grieving process because the life you once knew is gone. The person you used to be is gone. But the last stage of grief is acceptance. When you accept that you are chronically ill, the energy you used to exert fighting with yourself can be spent fighting for yourself... and slowly, everything else falls into place.* TRISHA

# Glossary

**Acupressure** involves deep pressure massage at points along the body's meridians (imaginary lines) through which energy flows.

**Acupuncture** is a means of Chinese medicine practiced for more than 3,000 years. Thin needles are inserted at points along meridians (imaginary lines) through which energy flows. It is used for pain relief.

**Activity management** is a way for people to manage their symptoms by learning to analyze and plan activities so that they can achieve more at home, at work, and at leisure.

**Aerobic exercise** is activity designed to increase the body's oxygen consumption.

**Aerobic threshold** is the heart rate during exercise at which a training effect will be achieved, usually described as being halfway between the resting heart rate and the maximum heart rate.

**Antidepressants** are medications used to relieve depression. There are different classes of antidepressants—for example, selective serotonin reuptake inhibitors (SSRIs) such as Prozac that increase the level of the neurotransmitter serotonin, which affects mood.

**Biofeedback** is a method of treatment that uses monitors to provide feedback to patients regarding physiological information such as heart rate, blood pressure, skin temperature, and muscle tension, of which they are normally unaware.

**Biomarker** is a chemical, typically a protein, found in the blood that is linked to the presence of a disease.

**Chinese medicine (traditional or TCM)** is the ancient system of health care from China based on the concept of balanced Qi (pronounced "chee"), or vital energy believed to flow throughout the body. Qi is proposed to regulate a person's spiritual, emotional, mental, and physical balance. It is supposed to be influenced by the opposing forces of yin (negative energy) and yang (positive energy). Disease is said to result from the disruption of the flow of Qi and the imbalance of yin and yang. TCM consists of herbal and nutritional therapy, restorative physical exercises, meditation, acupuncture, and remedial massage.

**Cognitive-behavioral therapy (CBT)** is a psychological ("talking") treatment that looks at how a person's thoughts, beliefs, behavior, and physical symptoms all fit together. CBT can help people feel more in control of their symptoms and to understand how their behavior can affect the condition, such as if they tend to "overdo" things on days when they are feeling a bit better. It does not mean that health care professionals think the person's symptoms are "in their head" or "made up"—it is used to help in many other illnesses such as cancer, heart problems, and diabetes.

**Cognitive dysfunction** is impairment in short-term memory or thinking ability with the feeling of "being in a fog."

**Complementary and alternative medicine (CAM)** represents a group of diverse medical and health care systems and/or practices that are not generally considered part of conventional medicine.

**Cortisol** is the body's primary stress hormone secreted by the adrenal glands into the blood. Cortisol reduces the actions of the immune system. Studies show that people with CFS and fibromyalgia have low cortisol levels, which could be why it is difficult for patients to deal with stress, infection, or exertion.

**Deconditioning** is loss of muscle mass and strength because of inactivity.

**Depression** is a state of mind characterized by sadness.

**Disease** is a sickness. The term refers to a condition when a structural or functional change in the body's tissues or organs has been identified.

**Disorder** is an ailment or an abnormal health condition.

**Endocrine system** is a system of glands, which secretes various hormones directly into the bloodstream to regulate the body.

**Exercise** is any kind of physical activity, including general everyday tasks, for example, brushing hair or getting dressed, sitting up in bed, and walking.

**Energy conservation** is a process of saving energy and better distributing the energy one has over the time one needs to use it.

**Flare or flare-up** is a term used to describe times when the disease or condition is worse.

**Fukuda**, named after CFS researcher Keiji Fukuda in 1994, is the research or case definition of CFS widely used in the United States to diagnose the illness.

**Genetic expression** refers to the process of how genetic instructions contained in your genes flows through to the production of a protein.

**Graded exercise therapy** is an approach for managing CFS that involves planned increases in activity or exercise, working toward goals that are important for the person with CFS. The first step is to help stabilize the amount of activity a person can do, and then a manageable level of exercise is added. This is gradually increased toward aerobic exercise if and when the person is able, aiming toward recovery.

**Homeopathy** is a type of medicine based on Dr. Samuel Hahnemann's theory that certain remedies stimulate the body's own immune and defense system to initiate the healing process. The practitioner prescribes individualized treatments based on the person's physical, emotional, and mental symptoms.

**Hypothalamic–pituitary–adrenal (HPA) axis** is one of the main brain-hormonal stress response axes, that is, places where brain function and hormonal function are coordinated in response to stress.

**Illness** refers to sickness or poor health. Diagnosis of an illness is typically based on the person's symptoms.

**Immune system** is made up of organs, cells, and tissues that work together to protect the body from disease caused mainly by bacteria, viruses, parasites, and fungi.

**Individualized education plan (IEP)** is a special educational plan developed by a school's special education team, the parents, and student to meet the student's academic goals and the means to achieve them, taking a disability into account.

**Inflammation** is a response to injury or infection that involves a sequence of biochemical reactions, causing fatigue, fever and pain, or tenderness all over the body. It can also cause local redness, warmth, swelling, and pain.

**Interstitial cystitis (IC)** is a chronic inflammatory condition that affects the bladder wall. People with IC have pain in the bladder and pelvic area, urinary urgency, and frequency of urination.

**Integrative medicine** is the practice that combines conventional medicine and complementary and alternative medicine (CAM) treatments for which there is evidence of safety and effectiveness. Integrative medicine was formerly called CAM or alternative therapy, which is misleading because the treatment modality that is integrated into conventional medicine has a body of research that demonstrates its safety and effectiveness.

**Irritable bowel syndrome** is a chronic, noninflammatory disease that causes abdominal pain and bouts of constipation and/or diarrhea.

**Massage** is a technique of applying pressure, friction, or vibration to the muscles to stimulate circulation, produce relaxation, and relieve pain.

**Meditation** is a technique that enhances relaxation and reduces stress. Through slower, deep breathing and mental focusing, the relaxation response can lead to more energy, better digestion, slowed heart rate, better sleep, and reduced pain.

**Melatonin** is a natural hormone normally produced in our bodies by the pineal gland to control our sleep cycles. It is used primarily to regulate our body's natural clock and address insomnia.

**Migraine** is a type of severe headache that may begin with spasms or constriction of the blood vessels in the head. It is often preceded by an aura, for example, flashing lights before one's eyes or an unusual odor, and accompanied by nausea and vomiting, pain, and sensitivity to light and sound.

**Myalgic encephalomyelitis (ME)** is another name used for CFS, for example, in Canada. Myalgic refers to muscle pain or tenderness. Encephalomyelitis means inflammation of the brain and spinal cord. Some researchers say that the E in ME stands for encephalopathy, which means altered brain function and structure caused by diffuse brain disease.

**Neurally mediated hypotension (NMH)** is characterized by a significant drop in systolic blood pressure (the top number in a blood pressure reading) of at least 20 to 25 mm of mercury when standing.

**Neuromuscular massage** is a therapy during which pressure is applied to specific muscles to increase blood flow or release tension or pain.

**Neurotransmitters** are chemicals that send chemical signals from one nerve cell to another across a space called a synapse. Examples of neurotransmitters include norepinephrine, dopamine, serotonin.

**Orthostatic intolerance** is an abnormal response to standing upright that can result in dizziness or fainting. It is related to low blood volume.

**Pacing** means trying to balance rest and activity to avoid making fatigue and other symptoms worse. Pacing strategies include setting activity limits, reducing activity levels, taking daily planned rests regardless of how the person is feeling, switching among tasks, and keeping detailed records.

**Pathogenesis** refers to how a disease and its related conditions develop, specifically what happens on the cellular level to cause reactions that lead to the disease.

**PWCFS** refers to people with chronic fatigue syndrome.

**Peripheral neuropathy** refers to numbness and/or pain in the hands and feet.

**Physical therapy** includes methods of rehabilitation to restore function and prevent disability following injury or disease. It may include massage, heat and cold applications, and an individualized program of exercises.

**Postexertional malaise** is extreme, prolonged exhaustion, the result of a worsening of symptoms that follow any kind of physical or mental exertion (not necessarily from intense or strenuous activity). It is an inappropriate loss of physical and/or mental stamina compared with the levels of activity leading to it.

**Postural orthostatic tachycardia syndrome (POTS)** is characterized by an increase in heart rate of more than 30 beats per minute, or to more than 120 beats per minute during the first ten minutes of standing.

**Relapse** refers to the return of CFS symptoms.

**Relaxation techniques** are methods used to relax your body and can be used to help with sleep problems, stress, anxiety, and pain.

**Remission of symptoms** refers to the disappearance of the signs and symptoms of a disease. When this happens, the disease is said to be "in remission." A remission can be temporary or permanent.

A **retrovirus** is a type of virus that inserts its DNA (genetic material named deoxyribonucleic acid) into one's cell's genetic makeup.

**Social security disability** is a federal program that provides financial assistance to people with disabilities who have worked long enough and paid social security taxes. Children with disabilities such as those related to CFS may qualify.

**Stress** is the body's physical and emotional reaction to external events taking place around us and within us. Studies have shown that there are actual physical changes occurring in our bodies when we are stressed.

**Syndrome** is a collection of symptoms and/or physical findings that characterize a particular abnormal condition or illness.

**Target heart rate** is the number of heartbeats per minute that people want to reach during exercise in order to gain its benefit.

**Trigger (or tender) point injections** are injections of a painkilling medication, usually lidocaine, directly into a tender point to relieve pain.

**Trigger point therapy** is a therapy during which concentrated finger pressure is applied to "trigger points" to relieve muscular pain. The trigger points, according to Chinese medicine, are points along invisible meridians that mark the path of energy through the body.

**Yoga** involves the practice of physical exercise and meditation. It is used to produce deep relaxation without drowsiness or sleep.

# Resources

## CFS Blogs

*Fibromyalgia and CFS Blog*–from Adrienne Dellwo on about. com brings a constant flow of short blogs dealing with recent events and topics. http://chronicfatigue.about.com/b/

*Four Walls and A View*–Dominique Dekker communicates regularly on her battle with CFS. http://www.pugilator.com/

*Learning to Live with CFS*–an informative blog from a mother with ME/CFS who has two sons with the disorder. http://www. healthcentral.com/chronic-pain/guide-154363-75.html

*Osler's Web*–Hilary Johnson, the author of Osler's Web, "thinks out loud" and contributes her ideas about CFS. http://www. oslersweb.com/blog.htm?post=700212

*Patient Advocate*–a Father's insightful search for answers for his daughter. Informative, heartfelt and wide-ranging. Follow him as he goes to the conferences and talks to the researchers and physicians. http://cfspatientadvocate.blogspot.com/

*Phoenix Rising Forums*—contain a large number of blogs by CFS patients. http://forums.phoenixrising.me/forum.php

# CFS Web Sites

*about.com* is a resource for information about CFS and FM, including original articles, chats, and breaking news. http://chronicfatigue.about.com/

*The CFIDS Association of America* provides current information, links, and an access to articles previously published by the organization. They publish The CFIDS Chronicle and provide a free e-newsletter and a series of Webinars on various CFS-related topics. The association directly funds CFS research and advocacy efforts and provides information and extensive educational materials on CFS. http://www.cfids.org

*CFIDS & Fibromyalgia & Self Help* is a nonprofit organization offering low-cost online self-help courses and other resources for people affected by chronic fatigue syndrome (CFS) and fibromyalgia (FM). The program was created by executive director Bruce Campbell, PhD, who had CFS and was a former consultant to self-help programs for CFS at Stanford University Medical School. The Web site also provides articles, forms, worksheets, and online books. http://www.cfidsselfhelp.org

*Chronic Fatigue Syndrome and Fibromyalgia Treatment Forum* is a site where patients can discuss treatment options. http://www.chronicfatiguetreatments.com

*FM/CFS/ME RESOURCES* is a patient-originated Web site that provides support, education, up-to-date medical news, research, coping tips and treatments, and informational resources to people with FM and CFS/ME, the medical community, and all interested. There are Quick Links to health care providers and disability attorneys as well as how-tos on topics such as finding a health care provider, and finding or founding a support group. http://fmcfsme.com/cfs_pediatric.php

*Fighting Fatigue* is a Web site with easy-to-understand articles and many resources and links to blogs and message boards regarding CFS and other chronic illnesses. http://www.fightingfatigue.org/?cat=14

*Lyndonville News (Dr. David Bell)* offers support, advice, recognition, and information to persons with CFS, ME, FM, and related, difficult-to-define, illnesses. http://www.davidsbell.com/index.htm

*The M.E. Society of America* is an informative Web site focused on myalgic encephalomyelitis. http://www.cfids-cab.org/MESA/

*Parents of Sick and Worn-Out Children* is a privately maintained site devoted to providing direction and resources for parents of children with CFS/ME/FM. http://home.bluecrab.org/~health/sickids.html

*Phoenix Rising*, a chronic fatigue syndrome (ME/CFS) and neuroendocrineimmune (NEI) conditions Web site, provides information on CFS, research, and treatments by Cort Johnson, the creator who has CFS. http://phoenix rising.me/ Find the Bringing the Heat Blog aboutmecfs.org and the Phoenix Rising Forums (forums.aboutmecfs.org) there.

*Pro Health* is an educational resource for information and the latest news and research about CFS. www.immunesuppressport.com

## Government-Sponsored Web Sites

*Centers for Disease Control and Prevention (CDC)* provides general information on CFS as well as programs supported by the Center for Disease Control and Prevention. http://www.cdc.gov/cfs/

*National Institute of Arthritis & Musculoskeletal & Skin Diseases (NIAMS)* is a division (or institute) of the NIH, and is responsible for studies on FM. http://www.niams.nih.gov/

*National Institutes of Health/NIAID Fact Sheet* provides a variety of resources for persons with CFS/ME. http://www.niaid. nih.gov/publications/cfsreso.htm

*The National Library of Medicine link* connects to the National Library of Medicine, and a program to look up scientific articles at no charge. http://www.nlm.nih.gov/medlineplus/

*National Library of Medicine CFS Facts* is a compilation of articles on CFS, summaries, and interactive tutorials, provided by the National Library of Medicine in Bethesda, MD. http://www. nlm.nih.gov/medlineplus/chronicfatiguesyndrome.html

*The Office of Research on Women's Health (ORWH)* serves as a focal point for women's health research at the National Institutes of Health. The Web site provides information on the CFS Working Group and its programs that is helpful to researchers, health care providers, people with CFS and their families, and the general public. http://orwh.od.nih.gov/cfs. html

*US Department of Health and Human Services Chronic Fatigue Syndrome Advisory Committee (CFSAC)* provides advice and recommendations to the Secretary of Health and Human Services via the Assistant Secretary for Health of the U.S. Department of Health and Human Services on issues related to CFS. These include factors affecting access and care for persons with CFS; the science and definition of CFS; and broader public health, clinical, research, and educational issues related to CFS. http://www.hhs.gov/advcomcfs/

*US Social Security Administration* provides general information about social security, as well as more specific information on obtaining social security disability benefits. http://www.ssa. gov

For information about Social Security programs: www.socialsecurity.gov

To apply for disability benefits: http://www.ssa.gov/apply fordisability/

To apply for disability benefits for children under age 18: http:// www.ssa.gov/applyfordisability/child.htm

# CFS Organizations

*Association for Young People with ME* (AYME) represents young people with CFS written by staff or volunteers in the UK, unless noted. Provides information and support about CFS http://www.ayme.org.uk/

*CFS Solutions of West Michigan* is a non-profit organization dedicated to improving the lifestyle and well-being of people with ME/CFS by providing educational materials, patient advocacy, and support services through monthly meetings and special events. Visit the organization on Facebook at http://www.facebook.com/cfssolutionswm

*Co-Cure* is a patient-run information exchange, most notable for the "Good Doctors List" that provides names and addresses of local doctors who are willing to see persons with CFS/ME/FM. http://www.co-cure.org/

*International Association for CFS/ME (IACFS/ME)* is an international organization of professionals interested in studying both CFS and FM. The IACFS presents annual update meetings for patients, and a biennial international symposium. http://www.aacfs.org

*The Massachusetts CFIDS/ME & FM Association* provides information about CFIDS/ME (chronic fatigue and immune dysfunction syndrome/myalgic encephalomyelitis) and FM (fibromyalgia) for patients, their families and loved ones, and health care providers. It also provides a range of support services for patients, including physician referral, disability counseling, support group referral, and support through an information telephone line and e-mail best suited for state residents but may help others by referrals. http://www.masscfids.org/

*National CFIDS Foundation* is a nonprofit, all volunteer organization with the goals of furthering research and helping people with CFS/FMS and related disorders. The organization funds research and provides information, education, and support to people with CFS. http://www.ncf-net.org/index.html

*The National ME/FM Action Network* is a Canadian, registered charitable organization of volunteers reaching out internationally and dedicated to helping the medical, legal, and general public in spreading awareness for myalgic encephalomyelitis/chronic fatigue syndrome and fibromyalgia (ME/CFS and FMS) through support, advocacy, education, *and* research *and the* publishing of a quarterly newsletter "QUEST," which is included with an annual membership fee. http://www.mefmaction.net/

*NJCFSA, Inc. (New Jersey Chronic Fatigue Syndrome Association)* is a not-for-profit, tax exempt organization whose purpose is to support patients, disseminate reliable information, and promote research. It sponsors a wide range of activities, including support groups, newsletter, phone list, statewide conferences, informational helpline, and interfacing with the CFS community. http://njcfsa.org/

*P.A.N.D.O.R.A. (Patient Alliance for Neuroendocrineimmune Disorders Organization for Research & Advocacy, Inc., PANDORA)* addresses and alleviates issues and challenges that affect the quality of life of persons diagnosed with neuroendocrineimmune disorders such as CFS, Gulf War illness, and multiple chemical sensitivities or environmental illnesses and persistent Lyme disease. It has established the Coalition4MeCFS and the Coalition4Fibromyalgia to provide a place for professional organizations to collaborate and share resources. http://www.pandoranet.info/ and on Facebook

*The Vermont CFIDS Association* raises public awareness of chronic fatigue immune dysfunction syndrome (CFIDS), supports and advocates for Vermonters who suffer the debilitating symptoms of this and related disorders, and facilitates the education of patients, families, health care providers, and primary care physicians in order to validate and establish a recognized and acceptable protocol for the diagnosis and treatment of CFIDS. http://www.vtcfids.org/

*The Wisconsin Myalgic Encephalomyelitis/Chronic Fatigue Syndrome Association, Inc.* is a nonprofit corporation dedicated to assisting patients within the state of Wisconsin. Its purpose is to act as a clearinghouse for CFS information within the state of Wisconsin; to assist patients and their families; to encourage communication among agencies, institutions, and concerned individuals; and to promote research on the cause, cure, and ultimate prevention of chronic fatigue syndrome. It offers a quarterly newsletter, discussion forum, phone support, and more. http://www.wicfs-me.org/

# CFS Sites for Youth

*The Center for Pediatric Hypotension*, directed by Julian M. Stewart MD, PhD, in Hawthorne, NY, investigates, evaluates, and treats adolescents and young adults with orthostatic intolerance, including those with orthostatic tachycardia, syncope, and other forms of chronic orthostatic intolerance including the chronic fatigue syndrome. http://www.nymc.edu/fhp/centers/syncope/index.htm

*CFS in Kids* is privately sponsored by the Nemours Foundation, this site provides tips on coping with chronic illness in kids, specifically CFS/ME and FM. http://kidshealth.org/parent/system/ill/cfs.html

*CFS in Youth Home Page*, a project of The CFIDS Association of America's youth program, provides resources and support for children, adolescents, and college students with CFS and related conditions such as fibromyalgia, neurally mediated hypotension, and postural orthostatic tachycardia syndrome. It also provides information and support for family members, teachers, school nurses, pediatricians, and health care providers who assist them. http://www.cfids.org/youth.asp

*Young Adults with ME/CFS—Support* provides the choice of joining an online support group and/or getting major updates about CFS. http://www.facebook.com/pages/Young-

Adult-Patients-with-ME-CFS-Chronic-Lyme-Fibromyalgia-
etc/183809648306533?v=app_49497528

# Research Institutes

*The CFIDS Association of America (CAA)* is the largest funder
of chronic fatigue syndrome research outside of the federal
arena. Under the guidance of nationally known researcher
from the Centers for Disease Control, Scientific Director
Dr. Suzanne Vernon, the CAA funds laboratory and clinical
studies, strengthens collaborations with investigators glob-
ally, recruits new talent to the CFS field, facilitates proactive
communication within the scientific community to share
ideas, knowledge, and data regarding CFS, and is building
a repository of blood and tissue samples from CFS patients.
http://www.cfids.org/about

*DePaul University's Center for Community Research* led by
Leonard Jason, PhD, has worked to define the scope and impact
of ME/CFS worldwide. http://condor.depaul.edu/ljason/cfs/

*The Dr. A. Martin Lerner Foundation* supports the work of
Dr. Lerner in uncovering the viral pathogenesis and cardiac
problems in CFS. The Foundation's goal is to create a molecular biology laboratory to produce diagnostic tests for subsets
of CFS patients and a training center to provide instruction for
doctors to treat CFS. http://www.treatmentcenterforcfs.com/

*Enterovirus Foundation* was started in 2008 by CFS patient
Lisa Faust to stimulate research into enteroviruses after
Dr. John Chia's study found high rates of enteroviral infection in ME/CFS patients. http://enterovirusfoundation.org/
index.shtml

*HHV-6 Foundation*, begun by Kristen Loomis, Daram Ablashi,
and Annette Whittemore, funds research efforts and sponsors conferences designed to advance the knowledge of dif-
ficult-to-detect central nervous system viruses. http://www.
hhv-6foundation.org/

*The Nightingale Research Foundation (NRF),* located in Ottawa, Canada, was founded by Dr. Byron Hyde in 1988, and incorporated as a charitable organization to explore and understand myalgic encephalomyelitis and chronic fatigue syndrome (ME and CFS) and fibromyalgia-type illnesses. NRF has provided technical assistance to health care professionals and researchers, and information to help and encourage thousands of North Americans who are patients or have family disabled by ME or CFS. http://www.nightingale.ca/index.php?target=about

*Pain & Fatigue Study Center* provides an integrated approach to scientific research and patient care headed by Dr. Benjamin Natelson, MD, medical experts on chronic fatigue syndrome and fibromyalgia. This center, located in Beth Israel Medical Center, New York, NY, is dedicated to understanding and treating CFS and fibromyalgia and provides clinical trials for PWCFS. http://www.painandfatigue.com/

*SolveCFS BioBank,* established by the CFIDS Association of America, collects and stores a bank of biological samples (such as blood, buccal tissue, cells, and DNA) and clinical information at the Genetic Alliance laboratory facility from individuals with CFS and unaffected individuals aged 10 and older. The samples and information are used by approved researchers to identify biomarkers and explore the causes of, and potential treatments for, CFS. http://www.solvecfs.org/

*University of Washington Center for Clinical and Epidemiological Research (UW CCER),* focused on using innovative strategies to conduct research that is relevant to the health care and well-being of underserved populations, uses an interdisciplinary approach in examining unexplained clinical conditions such as chronic fatigue syndrome and fibromyalgia, and health disparities in American Indian and Alaska Native populations. Its Chronic Fatigue and Pain Research Program is directed by Dr. Dedra Buchwald, an internist and leading researcher in the area of chronic fatigue syndrome. http://depts.washington.edu/uwccer/cpcf-about.html

*The Whittemore Peterson Institute for Neuro-Immune Disease (WPI)* exists to bring discovery, knowledge, and effective treatments to patients with illnesses that are caused by acquired dysregulation of both the immune system and the nervous system, often resulting in lifelong disease and disability. Scientists from the Whittemore Peterson Institute (WPI), located at the University of Nevada, Reno, NV, and their collaborators from the National Cancer Institute and the Cleveland Clinic, have discovered a retroviral link to myalgic encephalomyelitis/chronic fatigue syndrome (ME/CFS). http://www.wpinstitute.org/index.html

## Online Publications, Courses, Support, and Blogs

John, J., & Oleske, J. (Eds.). (2002). *A consensus manual for the primary care and management of chronic fatigue syndrome.* The Academy of Medicine of New Jersey, The University of Medicine and Dentistry of NJ, The NJ Department of Health & Senior Services. View the online manual at http://www.njcfsa.org/Manual.pdf

Campbell, B. (2010). *Managing Chronic Fatigue Syndrome and Fibromyalgia,* A Seven-Part Plan. http://www.cfidsselfhelp.org/store/managing-chronic-fatigue-syndrome-and-fibromyalgia

Campbell, B., & Lapp, C. (2010). *Treating chronic fatigue syndrome & fibromyalgia an integrated approach.* Campbell, B., & Lapp, C. is a self-study course that offers a step-by-step management and treatment plan that PWCFS can create. Includes free worksheets http://www.treatcfsfm.org/index.html?PHPSESSID=5da9702569de61baf3eab405dfa4f9c2

*CDC CFS Toolkit* provides health care professionals information about CFS and how to diagnose, manage, and treat symptoms. http://www.cdc.gov/cfs/toolkit/index.html

*CFS Facts.org* provides a blog for PWCFS that also contains CFS news, conference transcripts, and research findings. http://cfs-facts.blogspot.com/

*Slightly Alive* is a blog for PWCFS. http://slightlyalive.blogspot.com/

*Self-Study Course for Professionals (CME)* is a course developed by the CFIDS Association, the CDC, and HRSA to provide reliable education on the diagnosis and initial management of CFS/ME. It provides CME/CE credit for physicians and medical professionals. http://www.cfids.org/resources/print-self-study-module.asp

*Wrightslaw* is an educational Web site that provides parents, educators, advocates, and attorneys resources and information about special education law, education law, and advocacy for children with disabilities. http://www.wrightslaw.com

## Media

*Invisible*, DVD by Michael Thurston and Rik Carlson, gives voice to a select group of Vermonters who are gravely ill, and until now, have been out of sight. You will hear first person accounts from Vermont neighbors as they talk about living with chronic fatigue syndrome. http://www.invisiblethemovie.com/invisible_movie.html

DVD or the Limited Edition Combo Pack: DVD INVISIBLE and the book that inspired the move, "We're not in Kansas anymore" by Rik Carlson. http://www.invisiblethemovie.com/invisible_movie.html

*Vermont CFIDS Association.* http://www.vtcfids.org

*I Remember Me* by Kim Snyder is the first nationally released film about chronic fatigue syndrome. In this informative documentary about CFS, Snyder chronicles her own struggle with CFS and those of others. She interviews medical professionals and Olympic gold medalist Michelle Akers whose career was almost destroyed by CFS. http://www.cduniverse.com/search/xx/movie/pid/6730011/a/I+Remember+Me.htm

## Support for Caregivers

*caregiver-connect.ca* is a Web site that offers information and support for caregivers of CFS and other chronic illnesses. http://www.caregiver-connect.ca/en-US/Pages/Home.aspx

*CFS-CARE* is an Internet discussion group for caregivers of PWCFS and other chronic illnesses. Here topics discussed include emotional support, communication, research, diagnosis and treatment, related illnesses, support mechanisms, community, and humor. http://cfscare.com/default.htm

*National Center on Caregiving (NCC)*, established in 2001 as a program of Family Caregiver Alliance, the National Center on Caregiving (NCC), works to advance the development of policies and programs for caregivers in every state in the country. Uniting research, public policy and services, the NCC serves as a central source of information on caregiving and long-term care issues for policy makers, service providers, media, funders and family caregivers throughout the country. NCC provides the Family Care Navigator, a state-by-state online guide to help families locate government, nonprofit, and private caregiver support programs. It also provides caregiver information and assistance to identify resources and services for families and caregivers nationwide, educational and caregiver training programs, and more. http://www.caregiver.org/caregiver/jsp/content_node.jsp?nodeid=368

## Video Link

Rural NY Town Becomes Chronic Fatigue Laboratory 3/4/2011
Nearly 25 years after the "Lyndonville outbreak" of chronic fatigue syndrome, a controversy is brewing among scientists over what causes the illness. A small-town doctor hopes his patients will help provide the answer. WSJ's Jason Bellini reports. http://online.wsj.com/video/rural-ny-town-becomes-chronic-fatigue-laboratory/D80B17A7-B6C5-4B33-8356-F92C8751A93F.html

# Video Sources

*ME-CFS Knowledge Center* provides a variety of resources from around the world including a large video library of broadcast news, governmental hearings, medical lectures. http://www.cfsknowledgecenter.com/

*The ME/CFS Worldwide Patient Alliance* provides the latest news about CFS as well as videos and chats. http://mcwpa.org/ To participate in live video chat, instant messaging, forums and blogs with ME/CFS patients and medical experts from around the world, go to http://www.me-cfscommunity.com

# Fee Organizations

*The National Organization of Social Security Claimants' Representatives (NOSSCR)* is an association of more than 4,000 attorneys and other advocates who represent Social Security and Supplemental Security Income claimants. NOSSCR provides representation for claimants and advocates for beneficial change in the disability determination and adjudication process. http://condor.depaul.edu/ljason/cfs/

# Resources for Patient Medication Assistance Programs

For those who qualify, there are medication assistance programs available.

*BenefitsCheckupRx* provides people who are 55 or older with a confidential, personalized report of public and private programs that offer free or low-cost prescription drugs, health care, utilities, and other essential services. http://www.benefitscheckup.org

*Free Medicine Program* helps you cut through the red tape of applying for enrollment in patient assistance programs. www.freemedicineprogram.com

*Helping Patients* is an interactive Web site sponsored by PhRMA and 48 member companies to help patients and providers find patient assistance programs. http://www.helpingpatients.org

*Medicare* Web site provides a confidential online questionnaire to determine your eligibility for government programs. www.medicare.gov/AssistancePrograms or, based on the information you enter, the site searches for programs in your state or assistance programs for medications. www.medicare.gov/Prescription/Home.asp

*RxAssist: Volunteers in Health Care* is a national program supported by the Robert Wood Johnson Foundation. It offers an information packet that patients can download for prescription assistance. The database allows health care providers to search for patient assistance programs. There is a link to a list of state drug programs. www.rxassist.com

*RxHope* is a free, online resource to research patient assistance programs for more than 1,000 medications that provides an online application. Sponsored by PhRMA, the drug industry association, located in Hackettstown, NJ. http://www.rxhope.com

# Bibliography

## Chapter 1

CFIDS Association of America Commends AABB for Addressing Public Health Concerns. *International organization issues guidelines for blood donations by people with chronic fatigue syndrome.* Retrieved from http://www.cfids.org/xmrv/aabb-statement-june10.asp

CFIDS Association of America. *Diagnosis viruses.* Retrieved from http://www.cfids.org/about-cfids/viruses.asp

CFS Name Change Committee. Retrieved from http://www.cfs-healing.info/name-change.htm

Dellwo, A. *Epstein-Barr virus.* About.com Guide. Retrieved from http://chronicfatigue.about.com/od/cfsglossary/g/EBV.htm

Hickie, I., Davenport, T., Wakefield, D., et al. (2006, September 16). Post-infective and chronic fatigue syndromes precipitated by viral and nonviral pathogens: prospective cohort study.

*British Medical Journal, 333*(7568), 575. Retrieved from http://www.bmj.com/cgi/content/full/333/7568/575

Jason, L. A., Jordan, K., Miike, T., et al. (2006). *Pediatric case definition for ME and CFS.* Retrieved from http://www.iacfsme.org/Portals/o/pdf/pediatriccasedefinitionshort.pdf

Jason, L., Richman, J., Porter, N., & Benton, M. (2010). *Why the name of an illness is of importance.* IACFS/ME. Retrieved from http://www.iacfsme.org/WhytheNameof AnIllnessisofImportance/tabid/100/Default.aspx

Kamaroff., A. (2010). *The viral connection.* CFIDS Association of America Webinar. Retrieved from http://www.cfids.org/webinar/slides-091610.pdf

Kerr, J. (2008). Seven genomic subtypes of chronic fatigue syndrome/myalgic encephalomyelitis (CFS/ME): a detailed analysis of gene networks and clinical phenotypes. *Journal of Clinical Pathology, 61*(6), 730-739.

Komoroff, A. *CFS & the viral connection.* CFIDS Association of America 2010 Webinar Series. Recording of presentation: Retrieved from http://www.youtube.com/solvecfs#p/a/u/o/hyWSNitU-PQ

Marcus, A. D. (2011, March 22). Unlocking chronic fatigue syndrome. *The Wall Street Journal: Health.* Retrieved from http://online.wsj.com/search/term.html?KEYWORDS=AMY+DOCKSER+MARCUS&bylinesearch=true

ME/CFS 101. *What is ME/CFS? Causes.* Pro-health. Retrieved from http://www.prohealth.com/me-cfs/basics.cfm

Moore, D. (2010, April). What is chronic fatigue syndrome (CFS) and how is XMRV related? *NJCFSA Journal,* 30-31.

Schutzer, S. E., Angel, T. E., Tao, L., et al. (2011). *Distinct cerebrospinal fluid proteomes differentiate post-treatment lyme disease from chronic fatigue syndrome.* Retrieved from http://www.plosone.org/article/info%3Adoi%2F10.1371%2Fjournal.pone.0017287

Shyh-Ching, L., Pripuzova, N., Bingjie, L., et al. (2010). *Detection of MLV-related virus gene sequences in blood of patients with chronic fatigue syndrome and healthy blood donors.* Retrieved from http://www.pnas.org/content/early/2010/08/16/1006901107.full.pdf

Smith, R. A. (2010). Contamination of clinical specimens with MLV-encoding nucleic acids: implications for XMRV and other candidate human retroviruses. *Retrovirology, 20*(7), 112. Retrieved from http://www.retrovirology.com/content/pdf/1742-4690-7-112.pdf

## Chapter 2

Aaron, L. A., Burke, M. M., & Buchwald, D. (2000). Overlapping conditions among patients with chronic fatigue syndrome, fibromyalgia, and temporomandibular disorder. *Archives of Internal Medicine, 160*(2), 221–227. http://www.archinternmed.com

American College of Rheumatology. *Fibromyalgia.* Retrieved from http://www.rheumatology.org/practice/clinical/patients/diseases_and_conditions/fibromyalgia.asp

Black, D. W., Okiishi, C., Schlosser, S. (2001). The Iowa follow-up of chemically sensitive persons. *Annals of New York Academy of Sciences, 933,* 48–56.

Brown, M. M., & Jason, L. A. (2007). Functioning in individuals with chronic fatigue syndrome: increased impairment with co-occurring multiple chemical sensitivity and fibromyalgia. *Dynamic Medicine, 6,* 9.

Campbell, B. *CFIDS and fibromyalgia self help: overlapping and related conditions.* Retrieved from http://www.cfidsselfhelp.org/library/overlapping-and-related-conditions

CFIDS Association of America. *Do I Have CFS?* Retrieved from http://www.cfids.org/about-cfids/do-i-have-cfids.asp

CFIDS Association of America. *Treatment: Medical.* Retrieved from http://cfids.org/about-cfids/medical.asp

CFS/ME Diagnosis FM/CFS/ME Resources. Retrieved from http://fmcfsme.com/cfs-diagnosis.php

CFIDS Association of America. *Diagnosis: multiple chemical sensitivity (MCS).* Retrieved from http://www.cfids.org/about-cfids/multiple-chemical-sensitivities.asp

Chronic Fatigue Clinic, Johns Hopkins Children's Center. (2010, June). *General information brochure on orthostatic intolerance and its treatment.* Retrieved from http://www.cfids.org/webinar/cfsinfo2010.pdf

*Comparison table of Rome II and Rome III adult diagnostic criteria. Rome III disorders and criteria.* Retrieved from http://www.romecriteria.org/criteria/

Dellwo, A. *Fibromyalgia, chronic fatigue syndrome and irritable bowel syndrome (IBS): Why do they go together?* About.com Guide. Retrieved from http://chronicfatigue.about.com/od/whyfmscfsarelinked/a/IBS.htm

Dellwo, A. *The fibromyalgia diagnosis expect lots of testing.* About.com Guide. Retrieved from http://chronicfatigue.about.com/od/diagnosingfmscfs/a/diagnosingfibro.htm (Updated March 16, 2011).

DHHS CDC CFS Toolkit for Health Care Professionals. *Diagnosing CFS.* Retrieved from http://www.cdc.gov/cfs/toolkit/index.html

DHHS CDC Diagnosis. Retrieved from http://www.cdc.gov/cfs/cfsdiagnosisHCP.htm

Endometriosis.org. *What is endometriosis.* Retrieved from http://www.endometriosis.org/endometriosis.html

Eustice, C. *Guide to temporomandibular disorders (TMD).* About.com: Rheumatoid Arthritis/Joint Conditions. Retrieved from http://arthritis.about.com/od/tmj/ss/guidetotmdtmj_5.htm

Fibromyalgia & Fatigue Centers, Inc. *Coping with multiple chemical sensitivity syndrome.* Retrieved from http://pages.leadlife.com/ViewEmail.aspx?company=chronicity&email=lsteefel@aol.com&campaign=232&fwKeyWord=Week+of+November+1st+2010&emailID=522&jobID=17860

*Fibromyalgia.* Retrieved from http://www.aapainmanage.org/literature/PainPrac/08_spring08.pdf

IACFSME. *Myths of CFS.* Retrieved from http://www.iacfsme.org/MECFSMyths/tabid/311/Default.aspx

Papernick, M. *CFIDS Association of America Webinar. Co-morbid conditions: the alphabet soup of CFS.* Retrieved from http://www.youtube.com/watch?v=Cz6AolE6kHM Slides of presentation: Retrieved from http://www.cfids.org/webinar/slides-102110.pdf

ProHealth Library. *Mayo finds strong indication of genetic link in IBS: a syndrome common to a large majority of CFS and FM patients.* Retrieved from http://www.prohealth.com/library/showarticle.cfm?libid=12012

Torrey, T. *When you can't get a diagnosis. Failure to diagnose.* About.com Guide. Retrieved from http://patients.about.com/od/yourdiagnosis//failurediagnose.htm (Updated 2009, February 27)

Underhill, R. (2002, Winter). Gynecological concerns in women with chronic fatigue syndrome. *The CFS Research Review.* Retrieved from http://www.cfids.org/archives/2002rr/2002-rr3-article03.asp

Vernon, S. *Comorbid conditions receive focus.* CFIDS Association of America. Retrieved from http://www.cfids.org/cfidslink/2008/070904.asp

# Chapter 3

Associated Content. *The psychological component of chronic fatigue syndrome.* Retrieved from http://www.associatedcontent.com/article/191768/the_psychological_component_of_chronic.html

Bateman, L. (2007, May). Tips and travails of treatment. NJCFSA Fall 2006 Conference Coverage. *New Jersey Chronic Fatigue Syndrome Association Newsletter,* 1–9.

Berne, K. (1995). *Running on empty: the complete guide to CFS (CFIDS).* Alameda, CA: Hunter House; 57–60.

Berne, K. (1997). *CFS/FM symptom checklist.* LivingWithIllness. com Retrieved from http://www.anapsid.org/cnd/files/bernechecklist.pdf

CDC. *Chronic fatigue syndrome symptoms.* Retrieved from http://www.cdc.gov/cfs/general/symptoms/index.html

CFIDS Association of America. Medical provider information. CFS of Depression. Retrieved from http://www.cfids.
org/resources/provider-info-1.asp, Retrieved from http://
www.suite101.com/article.cfm/depression_women/110473#
ixzzovg4DCEJI

CFIDS Association of America. *Treatment: Medical.* Retrieved
from http://cfids.org/about-cfids/medical.asp

CFIDS Association of America. *Unraveling post-exertional malaise.* Retrieved from http://www.cfids.org/cfidslink/2010/
060204.asp

*CFS/ME symptoms and general information.* Retrieved
from http://www.ei-resource.org/illness-information/
environmental-illnesses/chronic-fatigue-syndrome-cfs-
myalgic-encephalopathy-me/

Dellwo, A. *Physical vs. emotional depression: FM & CFS.* About.
com Guide. Retrieved from http://chronicfatigue.about.
com/b/2009/05/26/physical-vs-emotional-depression-in-
fibromyalgia-chronic-fatigue-syndrome.htm

Dellwo, A. *Study: cognitive dysfunction in fibromyalgia.* About.
com. Fibromyalgia & chronic fatigue guide. Retrieved from
http://chronicfatigue.about.com/b/2010/11/17/study-cogni-
tive-dysfunction-in-fibromyalgia.htm?nl=1

Glass, J. (2006). Cognitive dysfunction in fibromyalgia and
chronic fatigue syndrome: new trends and future directions.
*Current Rheumatology Reports, 8*(6), 425–429.

Jason, L. (2009). Examining types of fatigue among individuals
with ME/CFS. *Disability Studies Quarterly, 29*(3). Retrieved
from http://www.dsq-sds.org/article/view/938/1113

Klimas, N. *Sleep, blood pressure, cognitive dysfunction.
Treatment options part I.* ME/CFS Knowledge Center, Inc.,
Expert Assistance Series. Retrieved from http://www.cfs-
knowledgecenter.com/ea4.php

McCaffery, M. (1968). *Nursing practice theories related to cog-
nition, bodily pain, and man-environment interactions.* Los
Angeles, CA: University of California at Los Angeles Students'
Store.

Robinson, S. *Results of a CFIDS association ME/CFS symptoms survey.* Fighting Fatigue. Retrieved from http://www.fighting-fatigue.org/?p=7732

Spotila, J. *Unraveling post-exertional malaise.* CFIDS Association of America. Retrieved from http://forums.phoenixrising. me/content.php?198-Unraveling-Post-exertional-Malaise-By-Jennifer-M-Spotila-J-D

Stewart, J. (2002). Dizziness in CFS. In J. John & J. Oleske (Eds.), *A consensus manual for the primary care and management of chronic fatigue syndrome.* Lawrenceville, NJ: The Academy of Medicine of NJ. Retrieved from http://njcfsa.org/Manual. pdf

VanNess, J. M., Stevens, S. R., Bateman, L., Stiles, T. L., Snell, C. R. (2010). Postexertional malaise in women with chronic fatigue syndrome. *Journal of Women's Health, 19*(2), 239-244. Retrieved from http://www.liebertonline.com/doi/abs/10.1089/ jwh.2009.1507

## Chapter 4

Acevedo, C. G. *Acupuncture treats chronic fatigue syndrome (CFS).* Suite 101. Retrieved from http://www.suite101.com/ content/acupuncture-treats-chronic-fatigue-syndrome-cfs-a289702

Bateman, L. (2010, November 11). CFIDS Association of America. *"DOC TALK": Communicating with your health care team about CFS.* Recording of Presentation: Retrieved from http:// www.youtube.com/solvecfs#p/a/u/o/E3y5hxJjj6s Slides of Presentation: Retrieved from http://www.cfids.org/webinar/ slides-111110.pdf

Bateman, L. *Ideas for finding a physician.* The National Fibromyalgia Doctor List. Retrieved from http://www.offeru-tah.org/findingadoctor.htm

Campbell, B., & Lapp, C. (2010). *Tips for caregivers.* Treating Chronic Fatigue Syndrome and Fibromyalgia. An Integrated Approach. Retrieved from http://www.treatcfsfm.org

*Chronic fatigue syndrome/myalgic encephalomyelitis (or encephalopathy).* National Institute for Health and Clinical Excellence. Retrieved from http://www.cnwl.nhs.uk/uploads/NICE%20CFS%20Guidance%20for%20Patients.pdf

CFIDS Association of America. *Treatment: choosing a healthcare provider.* Retrieved from http://www.cfids.org/about-cfids/choosing-a-doctor.asp

CFIIDS Association of America. *Choosing a healthcare provider fact sheet.* Retrieved from http://www.cfids.org/about-cfids/cap.pdf

Chronic Pain Association of Australia. *How to choose your healthcare (or pain management team).* Retrieved from http://www.chronicpainaustralia.org/resources/how_to_choose_your_health_care_team

FM/CFS/ME Resources. *Tips on finding a doctor.* Retrieved from http://www.fmcfsme.com/article_tipsforfindingdr.php

Mann, J., Brimmer, D. J., Boneva, R. S., Jones, J. F., Reeves, W. C. (2009). Barriers to healthcare utilization in fatiguing illness: a population-based study in Georgia. *BMC Health Services Research,* 9, 13. Retrieved from http://www.biomedcentral.com/1472-6963/9/13

ME/CFS 101. What is ME/CFS? *Causes.* Pro-health. Retrieved from http://www.prohealth.com/me-cfs/basics.cfm

National Institutes of Health, Medline Plus. *Talking with your doctor.* Retrieved May 19, 2010, from http://www.nlm.nih.gov/medlineplus/talkingwithyourdoctor.html.

National Institutes of Health, USDHHS. (December, 2008, D424). *The use of complementary and alternative medicine in the United States.* http://nccam.nih.gov/news/camstats/2007/camsurvey_fs1.htm

Share the care: how to organize a group to care for someone who is seriously ill. caregiver-connect.ca is a website that offers information and support for caregivers of CFS and other chronic illnesses. Retrieved from http://www.caregiver-connect.ca/en-us/communityresources/Pages/TakingCareofYou.aspx#section3

Steefel. L. *Chronic fatigue syndrome (ME/CFS) information for family, friends and caregivers.* New Jersey Chronic Fatigue Syndrome Association, Inc. (NJCFSA) Fact Sheet. Retrieved from http://njcfsa.org/caregiverfacts.htm

U.S. Department of Health & Human Services, Agency for Healthcare Research and Quality. *Reducing medical mistakes.* Retrieved May 19, 2010, from http://www.ahrq.gov/question saretheanswer/level3col_1.asp?nav=3colNav01&content=01_ 0_reduce

## Chapter 5

Bateman, L. *CFS and the exercise conundrum.* IACFS/ME. Retrieved from http://www.iacfsme.org/CFSandExercise/ tabid/103/Default.aspx

Bateman, L. (2007, May). Tips and travails of treatment. NJCFSA Fall 2006 Conference Coverage. *New Jersey Chronic Fatigue Syndrome Association Newsletter,* 1–8.

Blackman, G. How I gained hope and control: pacing for the bed-bound patient. Retrieved August 26, 2010, from http://www. cfidsselfhelp.org/library/how-i-gained-hope-and-control-pacing-bedbound-patient

Campbell, B. *Finding your energy envelope, part 2.* CFIDS and Fibromyalgia Self-help. Retrieved from http://www. cfidsselfhelp.org/library/finding-your-energy-envelope-part-2

Campbell, B. *Pacing for special events: slaying the dragon of post exertional malaise. Strategies for Special Events.* Retrieved from http://www.cfidsselfhelp.org/library/strategies-special-events

Campbell, B. (2001). *Ten keys to successful coping. Key 4: Nurture yourself with pre-emptive rest.* CFIDS and Fibromyalgia Self-Help. Retrieved from http://www.cfidsselfhelp.org/library/ 4-nurture-yourself-with-pre-emptive-rest

Campbell, B., & Cook, D. B. *Minimizing relapses: pacing yourself through the holidays.* CFIDS Association of America 2010

Webinar. Retrieved from http://www.cdc.gov/cfs/general/treatment/managing_activity.html

CFIDS & Fibromyalgia Self-Help. *The patient's guide to chronic fatigue syndrome & fibromyalgia 12: exercise, nutrition and chemical sensitivity.* Retrieved from http://www.cfidsselfhelp.org/library/12-exercise-nutrition-and-chemical-sensitivity

Dellwo, A. *Low motivation with fibromyalgia & chronic fatigue syndrome.* Fibromyalgia & Chronic Fatigue Guide. Retrieved from http://chronicfatigue.about.com/b/2010/09/29/low-motivation-with-fibromyalgia-chronic-fatigue-syndrome.htm

Dellwo, A. *Problems showering with fibromyalgia & chronic fatigue syndrome.* Fibromyalgia & Chronic Fatigue Guide. Retrieved from http://chronicfatigue.about.com/b/2010/11/16/problems-showering-with-fibromyalgia-chronic-fatigue-syndrome.htm

Jason, L., Muldowney, K., Torres-Harding, S. (2008). The energy envelope theory and myalgic encephalomyelitis/chronic fatigue syndrome. *AAOHN J, 56*(5), 189-195.

Lapp, C. W. *Treating CFS & FM: The stepwise approach.* CFIDS Association of America Webinar presented May 20, 2010. Slides with notes from Dr. Charles Lapp: Retrieved from http://www.cfids.org/webinar/lapp-slides.pdf

ME/CFS 101. *What is ME/CFS? Causes.* Pro-health. Retrieved from http://www.prohealth.com/me-cfs/basics.cfm

The National CFIDS Foundation. *CFIDS Treatment Options.* The National Forum. Retrieved from http://www.ncf-net.org/forum/lapp97.htm

The National Forum. CFIDS Treatment Options. http://www.ncf-net.org/forum/lapp97.htm

The Patient's Guide to Chronic Fatigue Syndrome & Fibromyalgia 12: Exercise, Nutrition and Chemical Sensitivity. http://www.cfidsselfhelp.org/library/12-exercise-nutrition-and-chemical-sensitivity

Smalley, D. (1997). *Energy conservation. Melissa Kaplan's* chronic neuroimmune diseases information on CFS, FM, MCS, Lyme disease, thyroid, and more. Retrieved from http://www.anapsid.org/cnd/coping/smalley.html

SportsMedicineDictionary.com *Aerobic threshold.* Retrieved from http://www.sportsmedicinedictionary.com/definition/aerobic-threshold.html

Spotila, J. (2010, September 1). Phoenix rising ME/CFS (chronic fatigue syndrome) forums. *Post exertional malaise IV: Power to the people.* Retrieved from http://www.cfids.org/cfidslink/2010/090103.asp

## Chapter 6

Beck, A. T., Ward, C. H., Mendelson, M., Mock, J., Erbaugh, J. (1961). An inventory for measuring depression. *Archives of General Psychiatry, 4*, 561-571.

Bell, D. (2005, January). Sleep in CFS. *Lyndonville News, 2*(1). Retrieved from http://www.davidsbell.com/PrintLyn NewsV2N1.htm

Bell, D. *"The first and central aspect of treating sleep disorders is good sleep hygiene."* Treating Chronic Fatigue and Fibromyalgia: Sleep Hygiene. Phoenix Rising. Retrieved from http://aboutmecfs.org.violet.arvixe.com/Trt/TrtSleepHygiene.aspx

Carruthers, B. M., & van de Sand, M. I. *ME/CFS a clinical case definition and guidelines for medical practitioners: an overview of the Canadian definition.* Retrieved from http://www.mefmaction.net/documents/me_overview.pdf

CDC. Course 1032: Diagnosis and Management. *Appendix: cognitive behavioral therapy for chronic fatigue syndrome.* Retrieved from http://www.cdc.gov/cfs/education/wb1032/appendix_c.html

CDC. (2010). Course 3151: A Primer for Allied Health Professionals. *Appendix: cognitive behavioral therapy for chronic fatigue syndrome.* Retrieved from http://www.cdc.gov/cfs/education/wb3151/appendix_c.html

CFIDS Association of America. (2010). *Contrasting chronic fatigue syndrome (CFS) and major depressive disorder (MDD).* Retrieved from http://www.cfids.org/resources/provider-info-1.asp

CFS/ME Working Group. (2002, January). Report to the Chief Medical Officer of the Independent CFS/ME Working Group [Electronic version]. p. 51. Retrieved September 25, 2006, from the Department of Health Web site: www.dh.gov.uk/prod_con-sum_dh/groups/dh_digitalassets/@dh/@en/documents/digi-talasset/dh_4064945.pdf

Cook, D. B., Lange, G., DeLuca, J., & Natelson, B. H. (2001). Relationship of brain MRI abnormalities and physical functional status in chronic fatigue syndrome. *International Journal of Neuroscience, 107*(1-2), 1-6.

Dellwo, A. Sleep Hygiene for Fibromyalgia & Chronic Fatigue Syndrome. *11 essentials of better sleep.* About. com. Retrieved from http://chronicfatigue.about.com/od/copingwithfmscfs/a/sleephygiene.htm

DeLuca, J. (2000, Summer). Neurocognitive impairment in CFS. CFIDS Association of America. *The CFS Research Review, 1*(3). Retrieved from http://www.co-cure.org/neuro.htm

Depression Guide. *Coping with chronic illnesses and depression.* WebMD. Retrieved from http://www.webmd.com/depression/guide/chronic-illnesses-depression

Erdman, K. M. *How biological abnormalities separate CFS from depression.* Retrieved from http://www.cfs-ireland.org/scientific/10.htm

FM/CFS/ME Resources. (2011). *FAQs about FM.* Retrieved from http://fmcfsme.com/faqs-fm.php#f22

Garcia, L. *CFS–an invisible and debilitating illness.* PANDORA. Retrieved from http://www.pandoranet.info/documents/editedLINAGARCIAMDCFSENGLISHarticleFinal_000.pdf

Jason, L. A., Najar, N., Porter, N., & Reh, C. (2009). Evaluating the Centers for Disease Control's empirical chronic fatigue syndrome case definition. *Journal of Disability Policy Studies, 20,* 93-100. Retrieved from http://www.prohealth.com/library/showarticle.cfm?libid=14824

Jones, D. E., Hollingsworth, K. G., Taylor, R., Blamire, A. M., Newton, J. L. (2010). Abnormalities in pH handling by peripheral muscle and potential regulation by the autonomic nervous system in chronic fatigue syndrome. *Journal of Internal Medicine, 267*(4), 394-401(8). Retrieved from http://www.ingentaconnect.com/content/bsc/jint/2010/00000267/00000004/art00006

Klimas, N. *Sleep, blood pressure, cognitive dysfunction.* Treatment options part I. ME/CFS knowledge center, Inc. Expert Assistance series. Retrieved from http://www.cfs-knowledgecenter.com/ea4.php

Lange, G. *Is CFS a brain disorder?* Retrieved from http://www.cfids.org/special/brain.pdf

Malouff, J. M., Thorsteinsson, E. B., Rooke, S. E., Bhullar, N., Schutte, N. S. (2008). Efficacy of cognitive behavioral therapy for chronic fatigue syndrome: a meta-analysis. *Clinical Psychology Review, 28*(5), 736-745.

McCleary, K. (2011). *Too big to fail.* Commentary on the PACE Trial. CFIDS Association of America. Retrieved from http://www.cfids.org/cfidslink/2011/lancet-study.asp

Podell, R. (2010). *Improving sleep quality despite fibromyalgia or chronic fatigue syndrome.* Dr.podell.org. The Podell Medical Practice. Retrieved from http://www.drpodell.org/improving_sleep_quality.shtml

Podell, R. (2002). *Sleep dysfunction in CFS.* CFIDS Association of America. Retrieved from http://www.cfids.org/archives/2002rr/2002-rr4-article01.asp

Spitzer, R. L., Kroenke, K., Williams, J. B. (1999). Validation and utility of a self-report version of PRIME-MD: the PHQ primary care study. Primary Care Evaluation of Mental Disorders. Patient Health Questionnaire. *JAMA, 282*(18), 1737-1744.

Steer, R. A., Cavalieri, T. A., Leonard, D. M., & Beck, A. T. (1999). Use of the Beck Depression Inventory for primary care to screen for major depression disorders. *General Hospital Psychiatry, 21*(2), 106-111.

Walker, V. (2005-2006). *Is sleep the root of CFS evil?* CFIDS Chronicle. CFIDS Association of America. Retrieved from http://www.cfids.org/special/sleep.pdf

White, P. D., Goldsmith, K. A., Johnson, A. L., et al. (2011). Comparison of adaptive pacing therapy, cognitive behaviour therapy, graded exercise therapy, and specialist medical care for chronic fatigue syndrome (PACE): a randomised trial. *The Lancet, 377*(9768), 823–836. Retrieved from http://www.thelancet.com/journals/lancet/article/PIIS 0140-6736%2811%2960096-2/fulltext

# Chapter 7

Bell, D. (2002). *David S. Bell, MD, on medications for chronic fatigue syndrome and chronic pain control.* Pro-health.com. Retrieved from http://www.prohealth.com/library/showarticle.cfm?libid=8206

Campbell, B., & Lapp, C. (2010). *Medications for sleep. Treating CFS & fibromyalgia.* Retrieved from http://www.treatcfsfm.org/submnu-Medications-for-Sleep-78.html

Dellwo, A. *Ampligen.* About.com Guide. Retrieved from http://chronicfatigue.about.com/od/treatingfmscfs/p/ampligen.htm (Updated June 28, 2011).

Dellwo, A. *Possible new chronic fatigue syndrome drug investigated.* About.com Guide. Retrieved from http://chronicfatigue.about.com/b/2010/08/25/droxidopa-chronic-fatigue-syndrome.htm (Updated 2010, August 25).

Dellwo, A. *The 7 genomic subtypes of chronic fatigue syndrome: Which type fits you?* About.com Guide. Retrieved from http://chronicfatigue.about.com/od/latestresearch/a/cfs_subtypes.htm (Updated January 26, 2009)

Harmon, M. (2005-2006). Clinical care for CFS. *The CFIDS Chronicle* (special issue), 48–51.

Immune Support.com. (2005). *Medications for chronic fatigue syndrome.* Retrieved from http://www.immunesupport.com/chronic-fatigue-syndrome-medications.htm

Kerr, J., Burke, B., Petty, R., et al. (2008). Seven genomic subtypes of chronic fatigue syndrome/myalgic encephalomyelitis (CFS/ME): a detailed analysis of gene networks and clinical phenotypes. *Journal of Clinical Pathology, 61*(6), 730–739.

Mayo Clinic Staff. *Chronic fatigue syndrome treatment and drugs*. Retrieved from http://www.mayoclinic.com/health/chronic-fatigue-syndrome/DS00395/DSECTION=treatments-and-drugs

National Institutes of Mental Health. (2011). *Alphabetical list of medications*. Retrieved from http://www.nimh.nih.gov/health/publications/mental-health-medications/alphabetical-list-of-medications.shtml

Phoenix Rising. (2004). *Treating chronic fatigue syndrome (ME/CFS): Ampligen part II–twisted history.* http://aboutmecfs.org.violet.arvixe.com/Trt/AmpHist.aspx

Phoenix Rising. (2004). *Treating chronic fatigue syndrome (ME/CFS) and fibromyalgia: anti-virals and antibiotic treatments.* Retrieved from http://aboutmecfs.org.violet.arvixe.com/Trt/TrtAntivirals.aspx

Phoenix Rising. *Treating chronic fatigue syndrome (ME/CFS) and fibromyalgia: a prescription for sleep.* (ME/CFS) Physician Recommendations for Prescription Sleep Medications. Retrieved from http://phoenixrising.me/?page_id=4809

University of Maryland Medical Center. (2011). *Chronic fatigue syndrome medications.* Retrieved from http://www.umm.edu/patiented/articles/what_drugs_used_chronic_fatigue_syndrome_000007_7.htm

## Chapter 8

Allen, J., and Meires, J. (2011). How to prescribe Tai Chi therapy. *Journal of Transcultural Nursing, 22*(2), 200-204.

Baranowsky, J., Klose, P., Musial, F., Häuser, W., Dobos, G., Langhorst, J. (2009). Qualitative systemic review of randomized controlled trials on complementary and alternative medicine treatments in fibromyalgia. *Rheumatology International, 30*(1), 1-21. Retrieved from http://www.ncbi.nlm.nih.gov/pubmed/19672601

Bateman, L. (2007, May). Tips and travails of treatment. NJCFSA Fall 2006 Conference Coverage. *New Jersey Chronic Fatigue Syndrome Association Newsletter,* 1-9.

Campbell, B. (2010). *Dr Lapp's recommendations on supplements.* CFIDS & Fibromyalgia Self-Help. Retrieved from http://www.cfidsselfhelp.org/library/dr-lapp's-recommedations-supplements

CDC. *CFS: treatment and management options alternative therapies.* Retrieved from http://www.cdc.gov/cfs/general/treatment/options.html#alternative

CFIDS Association of America. *Treatment: alternative therapy.* Retrieved from http://www.cfids.org/about-cfids/alternative-therapy.asp

CFS Toolkit. Retrieved from http://www.cfids.org/sparkcfs/2008/toolkit4.pdf

Dellwo, A. *Massage, rolfing & other bodywork: Are they effective fibromyalgia & chronic fatigue syndrome treatments?* About.com Guide. Retrieved from http://chronicfatigue.about.com/od/alternativetreatments/a/bodywork.htm?nl=1

Denison, B. (2004). Touch the pain away: new research on therapeutic touch and persons with fibromyalgia syndrome. *Holistic Nursing Practice, 18*(3), 142-151.

DiCarlo, G., Borrelli, F., Ernst, E., & Izzo, A. A. (2001). St John's wort: Prozac from the plant kingdom. *Trends in Pharmacological Sciences,* 1, 292-297.

Fibromyalgia & Fatigue Centers Inc. *Integrating alternative therapies into your treatment program.* Retrieved from http://pages.leadlife.com/ViewEmail.aspx?company=chronicity&email=lsteefel@aol.com&campaign=223&fwKeyWord=Week+of+October+4th+2010&emailID=501&jobID=10740

FM/CFS/ME Resources. (2009). *Supplements as fibromyalgia & CFS/ME treatments.* Retrieved from http://fmcfsme.com/article_supplementtreatmentsforfmcfs.php#1

Harmon, M. (2004, Spring). "Resources to lighten your load" in Rx for a lean budget. (2004). *The CFIDS Chronicle,* 6-9.

Healthcommunities.com. (2010). *Trigger point injections.* Retrieved from http://www.neurologychannel.com/tpi/index. shtml

Kam, K. (2009). *What is integrative medicine?* WebMD. Retrieved from http://www.webmd.com/a-to-z-guides/features/alterna- tive-medicine-integrative-medicine?rdserver=www.integra- tivemed.webmd.com

Mayo Clinic Staff. *CFS: alternative medicine.* Retrieved from http://www.mayoclinic.com/health/chronic-fatigue-syndrome/ DS00395/DSECTION=alternative-medicine

Mayo Clinic Staff. *Stress management. Yoga: tap into the many health benefits.* Retrieved from http://www.mayoclinic.com/ health/yoga/CM00004

Mayo Clinic Staff. *Stress management Tai Chi: discover the many possible health benefits.* Retrieved from http://www. mayoclinic.com/health/tai-chi/SA00087

ME/CFS Treatment by Modality. (2010). *Pro-health.* Retrieved from http://www.prohealth.com/me-cfs/modalities.cfm

Merkes, M. (2010). Mindfulness-based stress reduction for peo- ple with chronic diseases. *American Journal of Primary Health, 16*(3), 200-210. Retrieved from http://www.ncbi.nlm.nih.gov/ pubmed/20815988

Monzillo, E., & Gronowicz, G. (2011). New insights on therapeutic touch: A discussion of experimental methodology and design that resulted in significant effects on normal human cells and osteosarcoma. *Explore, 7*(1), 44-50.

Ong, J., & Sholtes, D. (2010). A mindfulness-based approach to the treatment of insomnia. *Journal of Clinical Psychology, 66,* 1175-1184.

Pro-health. (2010). *ME/CFS treatment by modality.* Retrieved from http://www.prohealth.com/me-cfs/modalities.cfm

Sensiper, S. *Alternative therapies for chronic fatigue syn- drome.* Beliefnet. Retrieved from http://www.beliefnet.com/ healthandhealing/getcontent.aspx?cid=13551

Smith, A. A., Kimmel, S., & Milz, S. (2010). Effects of thera- peutic touch on pain, function and well being in persons with osteo-arthritis of the knee: a pilot study. *The Internet Journal of Advanced Nursing Practice, 10*(2). Retrieved from http://www.ispub.com/journal/the_internet_journal_of_ advanced_nursing_practice/volume_10_number_2_11/article/ effects-of-therapeutic-touch-on-pain-function-and-well-being- in-persons-with-osteo-arthritis-of-the-knee-a-pilot-study.html

University of Maryland Medical Center. *Chronic fatigue syn-drome.* Acupuncture. Retrieved from http://www.umm.edu/ altmed/articles/chronic-fatigue-000035.htm

## Chapter 9

Bell, D., Floyd, B., Pollard, J., Robinson, M., Robinson, A. T. (1998). *A parent's guide to CFIDS.* Binghamton, NY: Hawthorne Medical Press.

CFIDS Association of America. (2002). *What is CFIDS in youth?* Retrieved from http://www.cfids.org/youth/youth. asp#CFIDS_affect_school_performance

Collinge, W. (1993). The path of self-empowerment. Chapter 5. Coping with your symptoms. In *Recovering from chronic fatigue syndrome: a guide to self-empowerment.* New York: Putnam/ Perigee. Retrieved from http://collinge.org/RecovCFSCh5.html

de Lourdes Drachler, M., de Carvalho Leite, J. S., Hooper, L. (2009). The expressed needs of people with chronic fatigue syndrome/ myalgic encephalomyelitis: a systematic review. *BMC Public Health, 9,* 458. Retrieved from http://www.biomedcentral. com/1471-2458/9/458

Fero, P. (1999). *An open letter to school personnel.* Wisconsin ME/ CFS Association, Inc. Retrieved from http://www.wicfs-me. org/wicfs-an.htm

IACFS/ME (International Association for Chronic Fatigue Syndrome/ME). Retrieved from http://www.iacfsme.org/ Home/tabid/36/Default.aspx

Johnson, C. (2008). *Taking stock: ME/CFS advocacy making headway.* Prohealth Library. Retrieved from http://www.pro-health.com/library/showarticle.cfm?libid=13518

Lupton, T. *Nurses can play a key role in CFS management*. The CFS Research Review. Retrieved from http://www.cfids.org/sparkcfs/nurses.pdf

Moore, R. C., & Albrecht, F. *Why children with CFS are often overlooked*. The Co-Cure Ring. Retrieved from http://home.blue-crab.org/~health/reb.html

New Jersey Chronic Fatigue Syndrome Association. Retrieved from http://www.njcfsa.org/ (Home page)

Phoenix Rising. *Making a difference in ME/CFS*. Retrieved from http://aboutmecfs.org/Adv/WhatYouCanDo.aspx

Silverman, M. (2007). *Marly's story. The importance of advocacy for CFS*. Retrieved from http://www.pandoranet.info/documents/Marly_Story.pdf

Social Security Ruling, SSR 99-2p. Notice of Social Security Ruling. Social Security Administration. Federal Register: April 30, 1999 (Volume 64, Number 83). Retrieved from http://www.cfids-me.org/disinissues/ssa0499.html

Social Security Online. (2001, April). *Providing medical evidence to the social security administration for individuals with chronic fatigue syndrome—Fact Sheet. ICN 953800. SSA Pub.* No. 64-063. Retrieved from http://www.ssa.gov/disability/professionals/cfs-pub063.htm

Steefel, L. CFS. *Information for family, friends, and caregivers*. New Jersey Chronic Fatigue Syndrome Association, Inc. Retrieved from http://www.njcfsa.org/wp-content/uploads/2010/08/3-4-NJCFSA-CarergiversMECFS20091.pdf

## Chapter 10

Bateman, B. *Family communication tips*. CFIDS & Fibromyalgia Self-Help. Retrieved from http://www.cfidsselfhelp.org/library/family-communication-tips

Bell, D. S., Jordan, K., & Robinson, M. (2001). Thirteen-year follow-up of children and adolescents with chronic fatigue syndrome. *Pediatrics, 107*(5), 994–998. Retrieved from http://www.cfids-cab.org/cfs-inform/Prognosis/bell.etal01.pdf

Collinge, W. Chapter 3. The recovery phase: when and why recovery happens. *Recovering from chronic fatigue syndrome: a guide to self-empowerment.* Retrieved from http://www.collinge.org/RecovCFSCh3.html

Fennell, P. *Four-phase model (FFPM). Overview.* Retrieved from http://www.albanyhealthmanagement.com/ourfocus_ffpm.shtml

Garcia, L. *CFS–An Invisible and Debilitating Illness.* PANDORA. Retrieved from http://www.pandoranet.info/documents/editedLINAGARCIAMDCFSENGLISHarticleFinal_000.pdf

Nisenbaum, R., Jones, J. F., Unger, E. R., Reyes, M., & Reeves, W. C. (2003). A population-based study of the clinical course of chronic fatigue syndrome. *Health and Quality of Life Outcomes,* 1, 49. Retrieved from http://www.hqlo.com/content/1/1/49

Thompson, D. *Ten tips to prevent a chronic fatigue relapse.* Retrieved from http://www.everydayhealth.com/chronic-fatigue-syndrome/tips-to-prevent-chronic-fatigue-syndrome-relapse.aspx

# Index

AABB. *See* American Association of
    Blood Banking.
Accommodations, schools and,
    103, 105
Acetaminophen, 78
Acetaminophen hydrocodone, 79
    Lorcet, 79
    Vicodin, 79
Acetaminophen with
    diphenhydramine HCl, 80
    Benadryl, 80
Activity to rest ratio, 53-54
Acupuncture, 41-42, 86, 90
Adderall, 79
Advanced practice nurse, as health
    care team member, 40
Advil, 79
Advil PM, 80
Advocacy, 97-101
    children, 101-103
    collaboration, 98

disability insurance benefits,
    108-110
education, 99
emotional, 100
family, 99
Individuals with Disabilities
    Education Act, 103, 104
organizations, 106-108
    Centers for Disease Control and
    Prevention, 107-108
    CFIDS Association of America,
    107-108
    International Association for
    Chronic Fatigue Syndrome/
    ME, 107, 108
    New Jersey Chronic Fatigue
    Syndrome Association, 107
    Patient Alliance for
    Neuroendocrineimmune
    Disorders Organization
    (PANDORA), 106

Advocacy (*cont.*)
   Sheridan Group, 107
   Vermont Chronic Fatigue
     and Immune Dysfunction
     Association, 107
  physical, 100
  schools, 103-106
Aerobic exercise, 53
Aerobic threshold (AT), 54
Aerobic yoga, 89
Age issues, 12
Allied health care professional, as
   health care team member,
   40-41
Alprazolam, 79
  Xanax, 79
Alternative therapies
  acupuncture, 90
  biofeedback, 89
  chiropractic, 92
  homeopathy, 90-91
  massage therapies, 86-87
  mindfulness-based stress
    reduction, 91
  osteopathy, 92
  physical, 93
  swimming, 93
  Tai Chi, 89
  therapeutic touch, 91-92
  yoga, 88-89
Ambien, 70, 80
American Association of Blood
   Banking (AABB), 13
Amitriptyline, 79
  Elavil, 79
  Sinequan, 79
Amphetamine, 79-80
Ampligen, 80
Anafranil, 79
Analgesics, 78, 79
Anesthesia, sensitivity to, 95
Anorexia, 18
Antiallergy agents, 79
  astemizole, 79
  loratadine, 79

Antianxiety agents, 79
  alprazolam, 79
  buspirone, 79
  clonazepam, 79
  lorazepam, 79
Antidepressants, 79
  amitriptyline, 79
  Endep, 79
  norepinephrine reuptake
    inhibitors, 79
  selective serotonin reuptake
    inhibitors, 79
  serotonin and norepinephrine
    reuptake inhibitors, 79
  serotonin, 79
  tricyclic, 79
Antihypertensives, 79
  atenolol, 79
  β-blockers, 79
Antihypotensives, 79
  fludrocortisones, 79
Antiseizure agents, 79
  carbamazepine, 79
  Neurontin, 79
  topiramate, 79
  valproic acid, 79
Appetite, 63
Armodafinil, 80
  Nuvigil, 80
Astemizole, 79
  Hismanal, 79
AT. *See* aerobic threshold.
Atenolol, 79
  Tenormin, 79
Ativan, 79
Australia, definition of CFS, 4

Back pain, 86
  acupuncture, 86
  lidocaine, 86
Baseline activity levels, 59
Beck Depression Inventory, 72
Bedbound patients, 59-61
  baseline activity levels, 59
  pacing, 59, 60

scheduling resting intervals,
    60-61
Bell, David, 113
Benadryl, 69, 80
Benzodiazepines, 81
β-blockers, 31, 79
Biofeedback, 89
Biomarkers, 9
    protein levels, 9
Bipolar disorder, 18
Blood donation, 13
    American Association of Blood
        Banking, 13
    viruses, 13
Blood pressure, 32
    disturbances, neutrally medicated
        hypotension, 22
Body positioning, 55
Brain abnormalities, 8
    hormone cortisol levels, 9
Brain fog. *See* cognitive
    dysfunction.
Bulimia, 18
Bupropion, 79
    Wellbutrin, 79
BuSpar, 79
Buspirone, 79
    BuSpar, 79

Calcium, 94
CAM. *See* complementary and
    alternative medicine.
Campbell, Bruce, 55
Canada
    definition of CFS, 3
    myalgic encephalomyelitis/chronic
        fatigue syndrome, 3, 6
    recognition of, 3
Cancer, 18
Carbamazepine, 79
    Tegretol, 79
Cardiologist, as health care team
    member, 40
Cardiovascular disease, 18
Caregivers, 47-50

CBT. *See* cognitive-behavioral
    therapy.
CDC. *See* Centers for Disease Control
    and Prevention.
Centers for Disease Control and
    Prevention, 107-108
    *CFS Toolkit,* 18-19
    definition of CFS, 4
    major criteria of CFS, 4
    public awareness campaign, 16
    recovery analysis, 114
    studies, 35-36
    symptoms of CFS, 4
Central nervous system, 29
Chronic Fatigue and Immune
        Dysfunction Association of
        America, 107
CFIDS. *See* chronic fatigue immune
    dysfunction syndrome.
*CFS Toolkit,* 18-19
CFS/ME. *See* Chronic fatigue
    syndrome/myalgic
    encephalopathy.
CFS/myalgic encephalopathy. *See*
    chronic fatigue syndrome/
    myalgic encephalopathy.
Chamomile, 80
Chiropractic care, 92
Chronic Fatigue and Immune
        Dysfunction Syndrome
        and Fibromyalgia Self-Help
        Program, 55
Chronic Fatigue and Immune
        Dysfunction Syndrome
        Association of America, 73
    questionnaire, 19
Chronic fatigue immune dysfunction
        syndrome (CFIDS), 2
Chronic fatigue syndrome (CFS),
        definitions of, 3-7
    Australia, 4
    Canada, 6
    Centers for Disease Control and
        Prevention, 4
    Fukuda, Keiji, 4-5

Chronic fatigue syndrome (CFS),
    definitions of (*cont.*)
  Great Britain, 4
  *Myalgic Encephalomyelitis/*
    *Chronic Fatigue Syndrome:*
    *Clinical Working Definition,*
    *Diagnostic and Treatment*
    *Protocols,* 6
  *Pediatric Case Definition for*
    *Myalgic Encephalomyelitis*
    *and Chronic Fatigue*
    *Syndrome,* 6
Chronic fatigue syndrome (CFS),
    ·naming of, 1–3
  CFS/ME Name Change
    Committee, 3
  CFS/myalgic encephalopathy
    (CFS/ME), 1
  Chronic fatigue immune
    dysfunction syndrome
    (CFIDS), 1
  myalgic encephalopathy/CFS
    (ME/CFS), 1, 3
  People with CFS (PWCFS), 1
Chronic fatigue syndrome/myalgic
    encephalopathy, 1, 2, 3
Chronic illness model, 115–117
  Fennell Four-Phase Model, 115
Claritin, 79
Clinoril, 79
Clomipramine, 79
  Anafranil, 79
Clonazepam, 79
  Klonopin, 79
Codeine, 78, 79
Cognitive dysfunction (brain fog),
    34–36
  medications, 35
  memory, 34
Cognitive-behavioral therapy (CBT),
    72–73
  effectiveness of, 73
Collings, William, 113
Complementary and alternative
    medicine (CAM), 41

Conserving energy, 55
  body positioning, 55
Contagious issues, 13
  blood donation, 13
  qualities, 9
Coping, 117–119
Comorbidity, 21
Crisis, Fennell Four-Phase
    Model and, 115
Cyclobenzaprine, 79
  Flexeril, 79
Cymbalta duloxetine, 79

Depakote, 79
Depression, 29–30, 66, 67–68,
    71–72, 94
  chronic fatigue syndrome vs.,
    67–68
  determination of, 72
    Beck Depression Inventory, 72
    Patient Health Questionnaire
      nine-item depression scale, 72
  medications, 68
  sleep, 68
Desipramine, 79
  Norpramin, 79
Desyrel, 80
  Trazodone, 80
Dextroamphetamine, 79
  Adderall, 79
Diabetes, 18
Diagnosis
  Centers for Disease Control and
      Prevention *CFS Toolkit*, 18–19
  challenges in, 17
  criteria, 26
  fatigue, 17–18
  hesitancy in, 16
  medication interactions, 23
  overlapping condition, 21–22
  related conditions, 21–22
  rule-out illnesses, 20
  second opinion, 22
  timeliness of, 16
Diagnostic questionnaire, 19

Diclofenac, 79
  Voltaren, 79
Disability insurance benefits, 3,
      108–110
  applying for, 109–110
  Social Security law, 108
Disease
  illness vs., 10
  syndrome vs, 8
Dizzy spells, 31
  β-blockers, 31
  blood pressure, 32
  orthostatic intolerance, 31, 32
  postural orthostatic tachycardia
      syndrome, 31, 32
Doxylamine, 80
  Nyquil, 80
D-ribose, 9

EBV. *See* Epstein-Barr virus.
Education, 30–32
Elavil, 79
Emotional symptoms, 29
Encephalomyelitis, definition of, 2
Encephalopathy, definition of, 3
Endep, 79
Endocrine system, interaction of, 2
Endometriosis, 18
Energy dollars (ED), 54
Environmental components, 9
  toxic exposure, 9
Epstein-Barr virus (EBV), 4, 9,
      15, 16, 66, 115
  Lake Tahoe outbreak, 4
  Lyndonville outbreak, 4
  mononucleosis, 9
Eszopiclone, 80
  Lunesta, 80
Ethnicity, 12
Evolution of CFS, 10–11
Exercise, 52–54
  activity to rest ratio, 53–54
  aerobics, 53–54
  baseline activity levels, 59
  energy dollars, 54

exertion levels, 56
  Lapp, Charles, 53
  medical consultations, 54
  monitoring of, 54
  post-exertional malaise, 53
  recording of, 57
  yoga, 55
Exertion levels, 56

*Family Practice Journal*, 29
Family relationships, 119–120
Fatigue, 25–26
  illnesses causing, 17–18
    anorexia, 18
    bipolar disorder, 18
    bulimia, 18
    cancer, 18
    cardiovascular disease, 18
    diabetes, 18
    endometriosis, 18
    fibromyalgia, 18
    Gulf War syndrome, 18
    hepatitis, 18
    hypothyroidism, 18
    lupus, 18
    multiple sclerosis, 18
  intensity of, 2
  post-exertional malaise, 26
Females, overlapping conditions
      and, 21
Fennell Four-Phase Model, 115
  crisis, 115
  integration, 115, 116
  resolution, 115, 116
  stabilization, 115–116
Fennell, Patricia, 115, 116
Fibromyalgia (FM), 18, 21–22,
      33, 65, 91
Flexeril, 79
Florinef, 79
Fludrocortisone, 79
  Florinef, 79
FM. *See* fibromyalgia.
Fukuda, Keija, 4–5
  case definition, 5

Gabapentin (Neurontin), 35, 79, 80
Gastroenterologists, as health care
    team member, 40
Gender population, 12
General practitioner, as health care
    team member, 40
Genetic links, 12
Genomic subtypes, 12
*Get Informed. Get Diagnosed. Get
    Treated,* 16
Great Britain, and definition
    of CSF, 2, 3
    Oxford criteria, 4
Gulf War syndrome, 18
Gynecologist, as health care team
    member, 40

Hatha yoga, 89
HCP. *See* health care provider.
Headaches, 26
Health care provider (HCP), 37–39
    allied health care professionals,
        40–41
    benefits of, 46–47
    communicating, 42–43
    complementary and alternative
        medicine, 41
    exercise, 54
    integrative therapists, 41–42
    journal keeping, 43
    medications, 43
    record keeping, 44
    referrals, 39–41
    search for, 38
    team members, 39–41
Hepatitis, 18
Herbs, 93–95
    side effects, 94
    St. John's wort, 94
High blood pressure, 79
Hismanal, 79
Homeopathy, 90–91
Hormone cortisol levels, 9
Hypotension, 22
Hypothyroidism, 18

IACFS/ME. *See* International
    Association for Chronic
    Fatigue Syndrome/ME.
Ibuprofen, 77, 79
    Advil, 79
    Motrin, 79
Ibuprofen with diphenhydramine
    HCl, 80
    Advil PM, 80
IDEA. *See* Individuals with
    Disabilities Education Act.
IEP. *See* individualized education
    plans.
Illness, disease vs., 10
Immune system
    abnormalities, 8
    interaction of, 2
Individualized education plans
    (IEP), 103, 105
Individuals with Disabilities
    Education Act (IDEA), 103, 104
    accommodations, 103–105
        individualized education plans,
        103, 105
Infectious agents, 10
Infectious disease specialists, 40
Integration, Fennell Four-Phase
    Model and, 115, 116
Integrative therapists, 41–42
    acupuncture, 41–42
Internal medicine, 40
International Association for
    Chronic Fatigue Syndrome/
    ME (IACFS/ME), 107, 108
    *Pediatric Case Definition for
        Myalgic Encephalomyeletis
        and Chronic Fatigue
        Syndrome,* 6
International Chronic Fatigue
    Syndrome Study Group, 4

Journal keeping, 43

Kabat-Zinn, Jon, 91
Kerr, Jonathan, 12, 76, 77

Klonopin, 79
Krieger, Dolores, 91
Kunz, Dora, 91

Lake Tahoe EBV outbreak, 4
Lapp, Charles,53
Lidocaine, 86
Lifestyle, balancing of, 61-62
Living with CFS, medications, 52
Lloyd, Andrew, 113
Loratadine, 79
    Claritin, 79
Lorazepam, 79
    Ativan, 79
Lorcet, 79
Lunesta, 80
Lupus, 2, 18
Lyme disease, 9, 13
Lymph nodes, 26
Lyndonville EBV outbreak, 4
Lyrica, 80

Massage therapy, 86-87
    myofascial release, 88
    rolfing, 87
    Swedish, 87
    trigger point, 87
MBSR. *See* mindfulness-based stress
    reduction.
McCleary, Kim, 73
MCS. *See* multiple chemical
    sensitivity.
ME/CFS. *See* myalgic
    encephalopathy/chronic
    fatigue syndrome.
Medical history records, 45t
Medical treatments, symptom relief,
    76-77
Medications, 33-34, 43, 68, 77-84
    ampligen, 80
    analgesics, 78-79
    antiallergy agents, 79
    antianxiety agents, 79
    antidepressants, 79
    antihypertensives, 79

antihypotensives, 79
antiseizure agents, 79
CFS specific, 78-80
gabapentin, 35
herbs, 93-95
interactions of, 23
muscle relaxants, 79
nonsteroidal anti-inflammatory
    drugs, 79
off-label, 78
psychostimulants, 79-80
sleep medications, 80
side effects, 80-84
sleep, 69-70
supplements, 93-95
Melatonin, 69, 80
Memory, 34
    loss of, 26
Mental relaxation techniques, 60
Migraine headaches, 26
Mindfulness-based stress reduction
    (MBSR), 91
    fibromyalgia, 91
Mirtazapine, 79, 80
    Remeron, 79, 80
Modafinil, 80
    Provigil, 80
Mononucleosis, 9
Motrin, 79
Moving medication. *See* Tai Chi.
Multijoint pain, 26
Multiple chemical sensitivity
    (MCS), 21-22
Multiple sclerosis, 18
Multivitamins, 94
Murine-related viruses, 107
Muscle pain, 26
Muscle relaxants, 78, 79
    antidepressants amitriptyline, 79
    cyclobenzaprine, 79
Myalgic Encephalomyelitis/Chronic
    Fatigue Syndrome, 1,2
    Clinical Working Definition,
        Diagnostic and Treatment
        Protocols, 6

Myalgic encephalopathy, 1, 2
Myalgic, definition of, 2
*Mycobaterium tuberculosis*, 10
Myofascial release therapy, 88

Narcotics,
    acetaminophen hydrocodone, 79
    codeine, 79
Nefazondone, 79
    Serzone, 79
Nervous system, 2
Neuroendocrineimmune diseases,
        106, 107
Neurologic symptoms, 29
Neurologist, as health care team
        member, 40
Neurontin, 79, 80
    gabapentin, 79
New Jersey Chronic Fatigue
        Syndrome Association
        (NJCFSA), 107, 115
NJCFSA. *See* New Jersey Chronic
        Fatigue Syndrome
        Association.
Non-narcotics, 78
Nonsteroidal anti-inflammatory
        drugs (NSAID), 79
    diclofenac, 79
    ibuprofen, 77, 79
    sulindac, 79
Norephinephrine reuptake
        inhibitors, 79, 80
Norpramin, 79
Nortriptyline, 79
    Pamelor, 79
NSAID. *See* nonsteroidal anti-
        inflammatory drugs.
Nurse practitioner, as health care
        team member, 40
Nutrition, 62-64
Nutritionist, as health care team
        member, 40
Nuvigil, 80
Nyquil, 80

Occupational therapist, as health
    care team member, 41

Off-label medications, 78
OI. *See* orthostatic intolerance.
Ormethylphenidate, 80
    Ritalin, 80
Orthostatic intolerance (OI), 31-32, 79
    water intake, 31
Osteopathy, 92
Overlapping Conditions Alliance, 21
Overlapping conditions
    comorbidities, 21
    diagnosis and, 21-22
    females, 21
    fibromyalgia, 21-22
    multiple chemical sensitivity,
        21-22
Oxford criteria of CFS, 4
    postinfectious fatigue syndrome, 4

Pacing, 55-57, 60
Pain management specialist, as
        health care team member, 40
Pain, 33-34, 77
    fibromyalgia, 33
Pain, medications, 33-34
    analgesics, 78
    codeine, 78
    multi symptom, 78
    muscle relaxants, 78
    nonsteroidal anti-inflammatory
        drugs, 77
Pamelor, 79
PANDORA. *See* Patient Alliance for
        Neuroendocrineimmune
        Disorders Organization.
Passion flower, 80
Patient Alliance for
        Neuroendocrineimmune
        Disorders Organization
        (PANDORA), 106
Patient Health Questionnaire nine-
        item depression scale, 72
*Pediatric Case Definition for Myalgic
        Encephalomyelitis and
        Chronic Fatigue Syndrome*, 6
Pediatric CFS, 12-13
Pediatric definition of CFS, 6-7
PEM. *See* post-exertional malaise.

People with CFS (PWCFS), 2, 10-11
Peterson, Phil, 113
Physical therapist, as health care
    team member, 41
Physical therapy, 93
Podell, Richard, 70
Population of chronic fatigue
    syndrome, 11-13
  age issues, 12
  ethnicity, 12
  gender issues, 12
  genetic links, 12
  socioeconomic background, 12
Post-exertional malaise (PEM),
    26, 27 53
  avoidance of, 57-50
  pacing, 55-57
Post-infectious fatigue syndrome, 4
Postural orthostatic tachycardia
    syndrome (POTS), 31, 32
POTS. *See* postural orthostatic
    tachycardia syndrome.
Pregabalin, 80
  Lyrica, 80
Primary care physician, as health
    care team member, 40
Protein levels, 9
Provigil, 80
Psychological symptoms, 29
Psychologist, as health care team
    member, 41
Psychostimulants, 79-80
  amphetamine, 79-80
  armodafanil, 80
  dextroamphetamine, 79
  modafinil, 80
  ormethylphenidate, 80
Public awareness campaign
  *Get Informed. Get Diagnosed, Get*
    *Treated,* 16
PWCFS. *See* People with Chronic
    Fatigue Syndrome.

Qi, concept of, 90

Record keeping, 44-46
  medical history table, 45t

Recovery
  CDC analysis, 114
  children,113
  chronic conditions, 116-117
  percentage of, 114
  sleep, 114
  time frame, 112-113
Referrals, 39-41
Related conditions, diagnosis and,
    21-22
Relaxation techniques, 60
Relief from symptoms, 76-80
Remeron, 79, 80
Resolution, Fennell Four-Phase
    Model and, 115, 116
Resting intervals
  mental relaxation techniques, 60
  scheduling of, 60-61
Rheumatologist, as health care
    team member, 40
Ritalin, 80
Rolfing massage, 87

*Science*, 13
Selective serotonin reuptake
    inhibitors, 79
  bupropion, 79
  mirtazapine, 79
  nefazodone, 79
Serotonin and norepinephrine
    reuptake inhibitors, 79
  Cymbalta duloxetine, 79
Serotonin, 79
Serzone, 79
Sheridan Group, 107
Side effects, medications and, 80-84
Sinequan, 79
Skin sensitivity, 30
Sleep, 68, 69-72, 114
  acetaminophen with
    diphenhydramine HCl, 80
  Ambien, 70
  apnea, 70
  Benadryl, 69
  chamomile, 80
  Desyrel, 80
  disturbances, 26

Sleep (*cont.*)
  doxylamine, 80
  eszopiclone, 80
  gabapentin, 80
  hygiene, 70-71
  ibuprofen with diphenhydramine
      HCl, 80
  medications, 69-70, 80
  melatonin, 69, 80
  mirtazapine, 80
  passion flower, 80
  pattern analysis, 70
  pregabalin, 80
  valerian root, 80
  zaleplon, 80
  zolpidem, 80
Social Security, disability
      insurance benefits and, 108
Socioeconomic population, 12
Sonata, 80
Sore throat, 26
St. John's wort, 94
Stabilization, Fennell Four-Phase
      Model and, 115-116
Stress, 64
Subtypes, CFS symptoms and, 76-77
Sulindac, 79
  Clinoril, 79
Supplements
  calcium, 94
  D-ribose, 9
  introduction of, 94-95
  multivitamins, 94
  Vitamin B12, 94
  Vitamin D3, 94
Swedish massage, 87
Swimming, 93
Symptoms
  CDC studies, 35-36
  central nervous system, 29
  common themes, 27, 32
  defining of, 7-8
  depression, 29-30
  diagnostic criteria, 26
      headaches, 26

  lymph nodes, 26
  memory loss, 26
  multijoint pain, 26
  muscle pain, 26
  sleep disturbances, 26
  sore throat, 26
  dizzy spells, 31
  education re, 30-32
  emotional, 29
  fatigue, 25-26
  immune system abnormalities, 8
  less common, 27
  neurologic, 29
  post-exertional malaise, 27
  psychological, 29
  recurrence of, 27-28
  relief from, 76-77
  secondary, 28-29
  skin sensitivity, 30
  studies of, 35-36
  unpredictability of, 25
Syndrome, disease vs., 8

Tai Chi, 89
TB. *See* tuberculosis.
Tegretol, 79
Tenormin, 79
Therapeutic touch (TT), 91-92
Topamax, 79
Topiramate, 79
  Topamax, 79
Toxic exposure, 9
Trazondone, 80
Treatment strategy, 14, 50
Tricyclic antidepressants, 79
  amitriptyline, 79
  clomipramine, 79
  desipramine, 79
  nortriptyline, 79
Trigger point therapy, 87
TT. *See* therapeutic touch.
Tuberculosis (TB), 10
  *Mycobaterium tuberculosis*, 10
Tylenol, 78
  Tylenol PM, 80

Valproic acid, 79
  Depakote, 79
Vermont Chronic Fatigue and
    Immune Dysfunction
    Association, 107
Vicodin, 79
Viral illnesses, 9
  Epstein-Barr, 9
Viruses, 13
  xenotropic murine leukemia virus-
    related virus, 13
Vitamin B12, 94
Vitamin D3, 94
Voltaren XL, 79
Voltaren, 79

Water intake, 31
Wellbutrin, 79

Xanax, 79
Xenotropic murine leukemia
    virus-related virus
    (XMRV), 13
XMRV. *See* xenotropic
    murine leukemia virus-
    related virus.

Yoga, 55, 88–89
  aerobic, 89
  Hatha, 89

Zaleplon, 80
  Sonata, 80
Zolpidem, 80
  Ambien, 80

# Northport-East Northport Public Library

To view your patron record from a computer, click on
the Library's homepage: www.nenpl.org

You may:
- request an item be placed on hold
- renew an item that is overdue
- view titles and due dates checked out on your card
- view your own outstanding fines

151 Laurel Avenue
Northport, NY 11768
631-261-6930